The 27 Simple Laws
For Diet and Exercise

An Easy to Read Guide to Living Healthy and Losing Weight

Author: Lee M. Spaziano

It's like an **Owner's Manual** for your body!

Featuring The Magic Formula Diet

The information in this publication contains the opinions of the author. The information in this book is in no way intended to be medical advice or as a substitute for medical consulting. The information should be used in conjunction with guidance and care of your physician. Consult your physician before beginning any diet and or exercise program, including those found within this publication. Consult your physician before beginning any weight loss program, exercise program, making important changes to your diet, or beginning use of any supplement. Supplements may have an interaction with your prescription drugs and or medical conditions, or pregnancy. Consult your doctor regarding your use of supplements before surgery.

The author specifically disclaims all responsibility for any liability, loss, or risk, personal or otherwise, that is incurred as a consequence, directly or indirectly, of the use and application of the contents of this book.

Copyright © 2014, 2019 Lee M. Spaziano

All rights reserved. This book or any portion thereof may not be reproduced or used in any manner whatsoever without the express written permission of the publisher except for the use of brief quotations in a book review.

Cover Art by: VisualArts.
Stock photography by: June Marie Sobrito, Julien Tromeur, Warren Goldswain, Olga Zaretskaya, and MacXever.

Ordering Information:
Printed by Kindle Direct Publishing, an Amazon.com Company

This book is available for purchase at:
  Amazon.com
  And other book stores

ISBN-13: 9781096862185

Printed in United States of America
Third Edition 2019

This book is dedicated to my beautiful wife Melissa, and to the best three kids a dad could have, Lynsey, Myranda and Alexander.

May you live long and healthy lives.

Good luck on your journey!

Lee

Table of Contents

INTRODUCTION 1

CHAPTER 1 - IN THE BEGINNING 4

CHAPTER 2 - PRIORITIES 6
   Law #1 - You cannot have good health unless good health is a priority. 6

CHAPTER 3 - GOALS AND DREAMS 9
   Law #2 - Write Down Your Goals. 9

GOALS WORKSHEET 19

CHAPTER 4 - SCHEDULING 20
   Law #3 - Schedule It! Put it on the calendar. 20
   Law #4 - Meal Preparation is the Biggest Saboteur of a Healthy Lifestyle. 21

CHAPTER 5 - LOGGING 23
   Law #5 - You Can't Manage What You Don't Measure. 23

CHAPTER 6 - WHY DO WE EAT? 26
   Law #6 - Will power alone cannot overcome your desire to eat. 26
   Law #7 - The Insulin Rollercoaster, nobody rides for free! 29
   Law #8 - You must control your body chemistry to control your appetite. . 31

CHAPTER 7 - METABOLISM 32
   Law #9 - You are in complete control of your metabolism. 32
   Law #10 - Breakfast really is the most important meal of the day. 33
   Law #11 - Eat a healthy snack or meal every 3 to 4 hours. 34
   Law #12 - Your body will cling to fat when in starvation mode. 38
   Law #13 - Dieting will eat up your muscles. 39
   Law #14 - Muscle Mass burns calories. 40

CHAPTER 8 - ICE AGE METABOLISM 45
   Law #15 - Simply Eating Less & Exercising More does not work. 46
   Law #16 - To lose weight, you must send your body the right messages. ... 47

CHAPTER 9 - LIFESTYLE CHANGE 48
   Law #17 - Permanent weight loss requires a permanent lifestyle change. . 48

CHAPTER 10 - WATER, WATER EVERYWHERE 50
   Law #18 - Don't Drink Calories! Avoid high sugar drinks. 51
   Law #19 - Drink Water. Drink 1/2 Oz for every pound of body mass. 52

Table of Contents

DIET 55

   CHAPTER 11 - EATING INTENTIONALLY 55

      Law #20 - You must eat intentionally to have a healthy diet & lifestyle. . 55

   CHAPTER 12 - FACT OR FICTION 58

      Law #21 - You must ignore all the diet misinformation. 61

   CHAPTER 13 - MACRONUTRIENTS 67

      Law #22 - You must have a balanced diet. Balance your macronutrients. 67

      Law #23 - Your calories should be 40% Carb, 30% Protein & 30% Fat. . 69

      Law #24 - A healthy diet has a low glycemic load. 75

   CHAPTER 14 - DIETARY WORKSHEET 81

   CHAPTER 15 - WHOLE FOOD 98

      Law #25 - Skip the Processed Food and stick to a Whole Food Diet...... 100

   CHAPTER 16 - READING LABELS 107

   CHAPTER 17 - THE MAGIC FORMULA DIET 110

EXERCISE 118

   CHAPTER 18 - STRENGTH TRAINING 119

   CHAPTER 19 - CARDIO 121

      Law #26 - Get plenty of exercise; both cardio and strength training. 128

CHAPTER 20 - SUMMARY 129

   Law #27 - Consistency is King. You can always find an excuse. 129

CHAPTER 21 - READING LIST 134

Introduction

Is this book right for you? If you know all about diet and exercise, macronutrients and micronutrients, and how to eat right, then this book is probably not for you. But you might want to buy a copy for all of your friends.

This book is for people who want to learn more about healthy living; how to have a healthy lifestyle through proper diet and exercise. I will show you the formula for success when it comes to eating right and living healthy.

Who will this book help the most?

You lost weight, but gained it all back.
Yoyo dieting happens because you go "on a diet" instead of changing your diet. Going on a diet can make you fatter. Being healthy takes permanent lifestyle change.

You don't understand nutrition and eating healthy:
There are all kinds of crazy misconceptions about diet and exercise out there. Fat is bad, carbs are bad, don't eat meat, avoid gluten. What the heck can you eat? This book will explain everything you need to know about how to eat right.

You are starting to notice your body ain't what it used to be:
Are you starting to get a little fluffy or maybe a little flabby? When you were young, you could get away with a poor diet. But now that you are getting older, years of eating processed food is catching up with you. For me, it was like somebody flipped a switch; one day I just started gaining weight.

This book is for anybody who wants to start eating healthily. If you want to make a change to a healthy diet and lifestyle but lack the knowledge to make it happen, this book is for you.

You have a poor immune system and get sick a lot:
Eating the wrong food will weaken your immune system and make you vulnerable to viruses, illness, disease, as well as a reduced quality of life. A healthy diet will keep you feeling great!

Skinny Fat:
Skinny fat is when you have a normal Body Mass Index, but a high Body Fat Percentage and a low Lean Body Mass. If you are "skinny"

but still a little flabby, this book can address your nutritional needs too. This book will help you tone up your body and look great.

Overweight or Obese:
If you are fat like I used to be, this book is for you. I will teach you the healthy habits you need for your new healthy lifestyle. You'll learn how to eat right, get appropriate exercise, and live a lifestyle that will allow you to reach your optimal weight for life!

Diet and exercise are a complete mystery to the majority of Americans.

We are constantly bombarded with television commercials telling us how we can have a perfect body with just 60 days of some exercise program or workout video. We are told to avoid carbs, avoid fat, don't eat too much of this or that. It seems today we are overwhelmed with media, information, and just plain noise on the topic of health.

How can we just cut through all the clutter and learn what really matters concerning our diet and health?

The 27 Simple Laws for Diet and Exercise is a no nonsense, easy to read guide to eating right and having excellent fitness and health. No matter what condition you're in today, following the simple laws in this book will help you live a longer, healthier life. This guide makes it easy for you to follow a few simple rules to be healthier. I'll walk you through the process.

Moreover, it will educate you on the topic of nutrition so you can make a lifetime of healthy decisions. You won't be blindly following another diet program. Instead, you will start to fundamentally understand what specific nutrition your body needs in order to feel great, be well, have longevity, and have a lean sexy body.

We discuss the healthy habits and lifestyle changes you need to make in order to be fit for life, everything from goal setting to time management. If your old habits have been failing you, it is time to make some new habits.

"If you keep on doing what you've always done, you'll keep on getting what you've always got." - *W. L. Bateman*

Introduction

Plus, the Dietary Worksheet helps you calculate your exact nutritional needs. As you go through the worksheet you will calculate your Lean Body Mass, Percentage Body Fat, Basal Metabolic Rate, and calories burned during activity, in order to find exactly how much of each type of food you need to eat every day.

Featuring the Magic Formula Diet. More than a weight loss program, this is a diet for life. Shed the fat you want to lose today, and then maintain your optimal weight and body composition for life by continuing to eat the correct amount of nutritious healthy food. It truly is like an Owner's Manual for your body.

Short on time?

If you're like most people, you're short on time, energy, and attention. You are so busy you barely have time to deal with life, never mind sit down and read a book. Don't worry about being too busy or having your A.D.D. kick in mid-book.

This book is short and sweet to accommodate your busy lifestyle. Each chapter gets straight to the point without a lot of fluff to fill the pages. I respect your time. Allow me to deliver this life altering information to you.

The book is broken up into three main sections. The first section has general information helpful for everybody. Section two focuses on diet, not dieting. Section three is all about exercise.

Applying the laws in this book will magically create more time in your day. When you are healthy and feeling high energy, suddenly everything else gets a little easier.

Good luck on your journey.

One last note... This is the sarcasm font. When you see this font, you know I'm being sarcastic.

Chapter 1 - In The Beginning

I started off much like you, struggling to live a healthy lifestyle, struggling with my weight, struggling to balance my work and family life with the need and desire to eat right and exercise. The problem was I simply didn't know how. I didn't have a knowledge base of how to live healthy. I had a bunch of old wives tales, urban mythology, and misinformation. My knowledge of healthy living was based on a montage of infomercials and miscellaneous comments at the water cooler.

You see, when I was younger, I could pretty much eat anything I wanted.

When you're young, you tend to naturally get a lot of exercise walking around the neighborhood, walking from class to class in school, cutting the grass, and what not. You tend to be on your feet a lot more. Plus you haven't yet been poisoned with years of toxic food, prescription drugs, and who knows what else.

As you get older your body just doesn't seem to work as well as it did when you were young. You're eating less, but still gaining weight. It seems like you're eating moderate portions and healthy selections, but year after year you add just a few more pounds. You don't have the energy to get out there and exercise.

Maybe you are drinking 4 cups of coffee a day. Maybe 6. Maybe even more!

Work, life, family, chores, you're just barely making it through the day.

How did you slip so far?

Trust me, I've been there too!

Starting in my early thirties my health started its decline. Before thirty years old, I was healthy, active, and strong. But after thirty, year by year, I slipped little by little. A few pounds gained here and there, work outs became fewer and further between. Next thing I knew I was fat!

In high school I was a healthy 175 pound male standing at 5'11". But suddenly at 36 years old I hit 242 pounds! Actually, it was not very sudden at all. Truthfully, I'd been watching, noticing the weight pile on for years.

In The Beginning

One day I bumped into an old friend. His words were, "Holy crap man, what have you been eating? It looks like everything."

Another time my wife and I bumped into an old acquaintance. My wife asked him, "Hey, I heard you lost 40 pounds?" He said "Yeah, but it looks like I just found it!"

It was obvious to me, and apparently everyone else as well, my health was slipping away and my weight was out of control. My wife didn't want to be married to a fat guy and I didn't want to be a fat guy.

So my journey began.

I read a ton of books. I've been to doctors, weight loss clinics, and even joined Weight Watchers. I've done the fad diets, I took the pills, and I injected the shots. I have been down those roads and discovered what works and what does not.

Use this book as a guide on your own journey. We'll talk about diet and exercise, weight loss, and muscle building. We will evaluate why we do what we do and how to make lasting changes in our lives and habits. Root cause analysis.

Chapter 2 - Priorities

Great news! About half the readers don't need to read beyond this chapter.

You have heard the expression a thousand times and a thousand ways...

> "I don't have time"
>
> "I'm too busy"
>
> "Ain't nobody got time for that"

The cold hard truth is that we all have exactly 24 hours in a day, 7 days per week, and 52 weeks per year. It's not about you having time to eat right and exercise, it is about you making it a priority in your life.

There are about a million things you could do today. You choose the things you want or need in your life. <u>You</u> set your own priorities.

Maybe you need to work to earn a living. Maybe you need to spend time with the family or help the kids with their homework. And the chores! That laundry isn't going to fold itself. If you get a moment of free time you just want to relax, catch up on that television series, browse the internet, or get on Facebook.

Well look, this is the simple truth.

Law #1 -
You cannot have good health unless good health is a priority.

I can't tell you what your priorities should be. Your mom can't force you to do it. You and only you can make the decision for good health, eating right, and exercise to be a high priority in your life.

Now is the time for you to make a decision; the proverbial fork in the road. I would argue that your health, happiness, and longevity are very important. Everything else is secondary because your health can and will impede those other things. Sure, going to the park with the kids is a high priority, but something you can't do unless you are well enough to get off the couch.

I recommend that right now, you make the choice to let healthy living be a high priority in your life. You make the choice to read this book and make the life changes necessary to live a longer, happier life.

If you're not ready to make that commitment to yourself you should just put this book down. There is nothing in this book or any other that can help you move forward without you overcoming this first hurdle.

However, if you are ready to make a change; if you are ready to let a healthy lifestyle be a priority in your life, please continue on. This book will give you the tools you need to be successful.

What does it mean to make healthy living a priority for you?

First of all, it takes a lot of effort. It is much easier to swing by McDonald's on the way home from work than it is to go home and cook a healthy meal. Reading labels, getting educated, exercising, these all take effort. You must accept the fact that this journey will take time and effort.

Something else in your life is going to need to be pushed aside to make room for your new healthy priority. So let's evaluate. Using the worksheet below, outline your top ten priorities. See if you can find room for healthy living (eating right and exercise) on the list of your top ten priorities.

My Top 10 Priorities

1. _____
2. _____
3. _____
4. _____
5. _____
6. _____
7. _____
8. _____
9. _____
10. _____

Did you find room in your life for healthy living? If so, you're ready to read this book. If not, don't worry. We all have different priorities. But don't complain about your health and fitness anymore because you made the decision.

You decide for yourself what you do and do not have time for in your life. Now it's time to live with that decision. Let's do it!

Chapter 3 - Goals and Dreams

Dream (drēm) *noun* 1. A series of images and thoughts going through one's mind. 2. A strong desire. 3. A fantasy.

Goal (gōl) *noun* 1. The end toward which effort is directed. 2. The state of affairs that a plan is intended to achieve.

We all have dreams, especially when we are young. I want to be President, I want to be rich, I want to be famous; all very respectable dreams. But what separates these dreams from real goals?

Goals require you to have a plan and be working toward the goal. Dreams you can do in your sleep, but goals require real life effort and real life work.

"A goal is a dream with a deadline" - *Napoleon Hill*

"If you don't know where you're going, any road will get you there."
- *Lewis Carroll*

So, what are your goals?

You should have written goals for all the different areas of your life. Get healthy, get rich, be happy; all good things, but not suitable as goals. Why? Because you need a specific goal with a specific date.

Law #2 -
Write Down Your Goals.

At the end of this chapter you will find a goal setting worksheet. Go through the worksheet and set your own goals. Here are some examples:

1. Get my body fat down to 18% by December 25th.
2. Earn 10% more money by this time next year.
3. Pay off my car by my next birthday.
4. Quit smoking by July
5. Give up drinking soda by next month.
6. Help my kids get honor roll this year
7. Run in a short sprint triathlon sometime next year.
8. Do a 5K run / walk next month.
9. Run a 14 minute mile by my next birthday.

All of these goals have a specific end date and condition. Things like "stop eating processed food" is a means to the end, but not really a goal.

Goals and Dreams

So what are some healthy goals that you might consider?

Goal to lose a certain amount of weight

Health professionals constantly debate the whole concept of losing weight. When you "go on a diet" to "lose weight" you are really reducing your total body weight. You want to reduce fat without reducing muscle, for various reasons to be discussed later. Considering that, is it really a good goal to "lose weight"?

Yes! If you are overweight or obese, yes. You do want to try to mitigate muscle loss, but in general you want to lose weight. If you want to be more acceptable in the health community you can call it "Getting Lean" or "Losing Fat", but let's keep it real here.

So then what is your weight loss goal?

The generally accepted method is to have a healthy BMI or Body Mass Index. *I can see my fitness pals rolling their eyes, but the doctors will love this topic.*

The problem with BMI is that it is a generalist approach which treats every body the same based on height and weight. Obviously a massive body builder is going to be much heavier than your average Joe. Fitness jocks will tell you to ignore BMI and use only Body Fat Percentage. However most doctors will agree with me, obesity is epidemic and BMI is the first line of defense. If you're an athlete, or muscular, BMI might not be for you. But for the vast majority of people, BMI works great.

Grab your calculators…

BMI = (Weight in Pounds / (Height in inches x Height in inches)) x 703

So if your weight is 210 pounds and you are 5'9" tall, your height in inches is 69".

BMI = (210 / (69 x 69)) x 703 = 31

Don't worry too much about this equation. You can always look up your BMI on a BMI Chart in this book or use an on-line calculator.

This is built into the TWB Smart Digital Scale, available on Amazon.com

BMI Chart

Height	90	100	110	120	130	140	150	160	170	180	190	200	210	220	230	240	250
6'4"	11	12	13	15	16	17	18	19	21	22	23	24	26	27	28	29	30
6'3"	11	12	14	15	16	17	19	20	21	22	24	25	26	27	29	30	31
6'2"	12	13	14	15	17	18	19	21	22	23	24	26	27	28	30	31	32
6'1"	12	13	15	16	17	18	20	21	22	24	25	26	28	29	30	32	33
6'0"	12	14	15	16	18	19	20	22	23	24	26	27	28	30	31	33	34
5'11"	13	14	15	17	18	20	21	22	24	25	26	28	29	31	32	33	35
5'10"	13	14	16	17	19	20	22	23	24	26	27	29	30	32	33	34	36
5'9"	13	15	16	18	19	21	22	24	25	27	28	30	31	32	34	35	37
5'8"	14	15	17	18	20	21	23	24	26	27	29	30	32	33	35	36	38
5'7"	14	16	17	19	20	22	23	25	27	28	30	31	33	34	36	38	39
5'6"	15	16	18	19	21	23	24	26	27	29	31	32	34	36	37	39	40
5'5"	15	17	18	20	22	23	25	27	28	30	32	33	35	37	38	40	42
5'4"	15	17	19	21	22	24	26	27	29	31	33	34	36	38	39	41	43
5'3"	16	18	19	21	23	25	27	28	30	32	34	35	37	39	41	43	44
5'2"	16	18	20	22	24	26	27	29	31	33	35	37	38	40	42	44	46
5'1"	17	19	21	23	25	26	28	30	32	34	36	38	40	42	43	45	47
5'0"	18	20	21	23	25	27	29	31	33	35	37	39	41	43	45	47	49
4'11"	18	20	22	24	26	28	30	32	34	36	38	40	42	44	46	48	50
4'10"	18	21	23	25	27	29	31	33	36	38	40	42	44	46	48	50	52
4'9"	19	21	23	25	27	29	31	33	36	38	40	42	44	46	48	50	52
4'8"	19	22	24	26	28	30	32	35	37	39	41	43	45	48	50	52	54

Weight in Pounds

Now that you've calculated your BMI, let's see what it means.

The BMI chart interpreted by the World Health Organization indicates that if you have a BMI over 25 you are overweight. A BMI above 30 means you are Obese.

Example Goal: Drop my BMI to 30 within 6 months and to 25 within 24 months.

Meaning	BMI
Normal weight	19–24.9
Over weight	25–29.9
Obesity I	30–34.9
Obesity II	35–39.9
Obesity III	≥ 40

Goals and Dreams

Goal to lose a certain amount of fat

A healthier alternative to losing weight is losing fat. We're talking about getting lean. If you are athletic or if you are "Skinny Fat", this is more for you.

BMI is easy, just look it up on the chart and you're done. But body fat content takes a little more consideration. Let's say you want to monitor your fat loss and your muscle gain, or suppose you just want to check that you are not losing muscle. You will need to know your Lean Body Mass and your Body Fat Percentage.

Lean Body Mass (LBM):
The weight of everything in your body excluding fat.

Body Fat Percentage:
The percentage of your total weight which is body fat. The weight of the person's fat divided by the person's total weight.

Healthy Body Fat Percentage differs in men and women because women typically have larger healthy fat stores in their hips and breast. Keep in mind (as we will discuss later) body fat is important; you will literally die if it were to drop too low.

Healthy Body Fat for Men
- Ages 20-39: 8% to 19%
- Ages 40-59: 11% to 21%
- Ages 60+ : 13% to 24%

Healthy Body Fat for Women
- Ages 20-39: 21% to 32%
- Ages 40-59: 23% to 33%
- Ages 60+ : 24% to 35%

If you want to get ripped to see killer abs and every little muscle striation, 8% body fat is what it takes. If you want to be a great runner, 17% or so should do nicely. If you just want to avoid death by cardiac arrest, 22% for men and 30% for women should be just fine.

	Men	**Women**
Essential % of Fat	2 - 5%	10 - 13%
Typical Athlete	6 - 13 %	14 - 20 %
Physically Fit	14 - 17 %	21 - 24 %
Acceptable	18 - 24 %	25 - 31 %
Obese	25% or more	32% or more

Guidelines established by the American Council on Exercise

How to Calculate Body Fat Percentage?

There are lots of different methods for calculating body fat percentage, each more or less accurate depending on your body style. There are wide variations in error for all of these methods. For example, at one point I used the Omron hand held Fat Loss Monitor and the Omron scale on the same day. The hand held device read 20% while the scale said 30%, clearly an unacceptable difference.

The two methods I like best are:

1. Hand held Fat Loss Monitor purchased on-line for around $20
2. Measuring tape and a calculator.

For Men:

Measure: Bodyweight in pounds

Measure: Waist circumference in inches at the belly button

LBM = (Bodyweight x 1.082) + 94.42 - (Waist Circumference x 4.15)

$$\text{Percentage Body Fat} = \frac{(\text{Bodyweight} - \text{Lean Body Mass}) \times 100}{\text{Bodyweight}}$$

For Women:

    Measure: Bodyweight in pounds

    Measure: Waist circumference in inches at the belly button

    Measure: Wrist circumference

    Measure: Hip circumference at the widest point

    Measure: Forearm circumference at the widest point

$$\begin{aligned} LBM = \ & \text{Weight} \times 0.732 \\ & + 8.987 \\ & + \text{Wrist} / 3.14 \\ & - \text{Waist} \times 0.157 \\ & - \text{Hip} \times 0.249 \\ & + \text{Arm} \times 0.434 \end{aligned}$$

$$\text{Percentage Body Fat} = \frac{(\text{Bodyweight} - \text{Lean Body Mass}) \times 100}{\text{Bodyweight}}$$

Or you can just use our built in feature in the TWB Smart Digital Scale, available on Amazon.com.

Example Goal: Drop my body fat percentage to 21% by Labor Day.

Example Goal: Raise my LBM to 120 lbs by New Year's Day

Goal to reduce resting heart rate

Resting heart rate (RHR) has long been considered the best measure of fitness. The more quality cardiovascular training you do, the lower your resting heart rate will be. Some elite athletes have a RHR as low 50 BPM, whereas a couch potato could be as high as 85 BPM. The lower your resting heart rate the better your overall cardiac health.

How do you improve your resting heart rate (RHR)?

Lots of High Intensity Interval Training (HIIT), cardio, or even walking can help. Any exercise that gets your heart rate into zone 1 or higher will get you going in the right direction. (We'll talk about heart rate zone training later)

How do you measure your resting heart rate?

Using a heart rate monitor or just a simple stop watch, take your pulse while resting. It is best to take your RHR first thing in the morning. Otherwise, you should be sitting resting calmly for at least 10 minutes. Caffeine, digestion, anxiety, and many other factors can increase your heart rate. Taking your RHR first thing in the morning eliminates these factors.

Example Goal: Drop my resting heart rate to 62 BPM by July 4th.

Resting Heart Rate Chart

RHR	18-25	26-35	36-45	45-55	56-65	66+
49	Athlete	Athlete	Athlete	Athlete	Athlete	Athlete
50	Athlete	Athlete	Athlete	Athlete	Athlete	Athlete
51	Athlete	Athlete	Athlete	Athlete	Athlete	Athlete
52	Athlete	Athlete	Athlete	Athlete	Athlete	Athlete
53	Athlete	Athlete	Athlete	Athlete	Athlete	Athlete
54	Athlete	Athlete	Athlete	Athlete	Athlete	Athlete
55	Athlete	Excellent	Athlete	Athlete	Athlete	Athlete
56	Excellent	Excellent	Athlete	Athlete	Athlete	Excellent
57	Excellent	Excellent	Excellent	Athlete	Excellent	Excellent
58	Excellent	Excellent	Excellent	Excellent	Excellent	Excellent
59	Excellent	Excellent	Excellent	Excellent	Excellent	Excellent
60	Excellent	Excellent	Excellent	Excellent	Excellent	Excellent
61	Excellent	Excellent	Excellent	Excellent	Excellent	Excellent
62	Good	Good	Excellent	Excellent	Good	Good
63	Good	Good	Good	Excellent	Good	Good
64	Good	Good	Good	Good	Good	Good
65	Good	Good	Good	Good	Good	Good
66	Above Avg	Above Avg	Good	Good	Good	Above Avg
67	Above Avg	Above Avg	Above Avg	Good	Good	Above Avg
68	Above Avg	Above Avg	Above Avg	Above Avg	Above Avg	Above Avg
69	Above Avg	Above Avg	Above Avg	Above Avg	Above Avg	Above Avg
70	Average	Above Avg	Above Avg	Above Avg	Above Avg	Average
71	Average	Average	Average	Above Avg	Above Avg	Average
72	Average	Average	Average	Average	Average	Average
73	Average	Average	Average	Average	Average	Average
74	Below Avg	Average	Average	Average	Average	Below Avg
75	Below Avg	Below Avg	Average	Average	Average	Below Avg
76	Below Avg	Below Avg	Below Avg	Average	Below Avg	Below Avg
77	Below Avg	Below Avg	Below Avg	Below Avg	Below Avg	Below Avg
78	Below Avg	Below Avg	Below Avg	Below Avg	Below Avg	Below Avg
79	Below Avg	Below Avg	Below Avg	Below Avg	Below Avg	Below Avg
80	Below Avg	Below Avg	Below Avg	Below Avg	Below Avg	Poor
81	Below Avg	Below Avg	Below Avg	Below Avg	Below Avg	Poor
82	Poor	Poor	Below Avg	Below Avg	Poor	Poor
83	Poor	Poor	Poor	Below Avg	Poor	Poor
84	Poor	Poor	Poor	Poor	Poor	Poor
85	Poor	Poor	Poor	Poor	Poor	Poor

Good Resting Heart Rate Chart: SportsScience.com

Goal C25K

Couch to 5K is a common training program used by beginner runners just getting off the couch. There are various programs to help you reach various goals.

Search online and you'll find lots of local races for all different levels of athletes. You can walk or run, completely up to you. Trust me; I'm a relatively slow runner. No matter your pace, there is a place for you at these events. At just about every race the winner finishes in 15 minutes, and the final finisher comes in at one hour and ten minutes. There are a wide variety of participants.

Nobody is judging you. To the contrary, large people get even more respect just for getting out there and doing the event. It is easy for me to show up because I'm physically fit (now anyway). An obese person really has to put in the extra effort to just show up. Mad props!

Example Goal: Be ready for and complete the Family Fest 5K Walk / Run in September.

Example Goal: Run 12 minute miles in the Find a Cure 5K in October.

It really does not matter too much what your goals are as long as they are right for you. Write them down and work the plan.

Goals Worksheet

Long-Term Goals (10 Years):
_____
_____
_____

Medium-Term Goals (5 Years):
_____
_____
_____

Short-Term Goals (1 Year):
_____
_____
_____

Most Important Goals
1. _____
2. _____
3. _____

What could get in my way?
_____
_____
_____

What actions do I need to take?
_____
_____
_____
_____
_____
_____

Career Goals
- Get a promotion
- Reach new level
- Learn a new skill
- Complete project

My Career Goals
_____
_____
_____

Financial Goals
- Pay off debt
- Emergency fund
- Set-up IRA
- Pay off car

My Financial Goals
_____
_____
_____

Educational Goals
- Financial Peace University
- Master's Degree
- Take a real estate class
- CE Classes

My Educational Goals
_____
_____
_____

Health and Fitness Goals
- Body Fat 18%
- Do a sprint triathlon
- Run/Walk a 5K
- Reduce resting HR

My Health Goals
_____
_____
_____

Misc. Goals
Misc. Goals
_____
_____
_____

Chapter 4 - Scheduling

Health and exercise is not something you just squeeze into your schedule. To be successful you need to schedule it intentionally. Put it on the calendar, block out the time.

Law #3 -
Schedule It! Put it on the calendar.

We all know what it's like. You're busy. Life is hectic and sometimes crazy. We all tend to procrastinate. Next thing you know, you skipped another workout or you ran out to grab a quick Chalupa from Taco Bell.

Guess what? Good intentions are not good enough. You <u>must schedule</u> your meals and workouts. Live Intentionally!

How to do it?

Eating:

First, let's consider meals. We are going to talk about what you should eat, when you should eat, and why you should eat, but for now let's just consider the intentional schedule.

When will you eat breakfast, lunch, and dinner? How about snacks? If you are anything like most people, you eat when you think you are hungry or when you can find the time. That's not going to cut it!

You can't just eat whenever you feel like and expect to have good results. Failing to plan is planning to fail. Don't schedule your meals around your life; schedule your life around your meals. Sure you need to be practical, but you also need to be working toward your goals.

You need to decide when to eat your meals and snacks. Put the meals on your schedule and stick to it. If the schedule is not perfect you can always make adjustments.

Meal Preparation:

You skipped breakfast and ate lunch at noon. You are just now getting home from work at 6:30 PM and you are hungry. Really hungry! You start to make dinner for yourself, but you just need a little snack to hold you over. How about an entire bag of Oreo Cookies?

Yeah, I did that. So what?

Shopping for healthy food and preparing healthy snacks and meals takes time. This is the number one diet killer. You want to eat healthy, but sneaking out for a chili dog is a lot easier than cooking up some vegetable stir fry.

We can all be a little lazy. Who wants to mess around in the kitchen when you could be watching American Idol?

You must plan out, shop for, and prepare your meals in advance. You should not be staring into the refrigerator asking yourself what you are having for dinner. Meals should be preplanned.

Law #4 -
Meal Preparation is the Biggest Saboteur of a Healthy Lifestyle.

Don't sabotage yourself and your new healthy diet by failing to plan for and schedule time for meal preparation. Plan your meals intentionally and prepare in advance.

Exercise:

When do you want to exercise? Before work? During lunch hours? After work? After dinner? Or maybe the answer is, "I don't know when I'll exercise. I just know I don't have time right now".

Most people have a real tough time trying to fit exercise into their schedules. In the morning you're tired and in a hurry to get the kids off to school, go to work, or just get out the door. It's too hot during the day or maybe you can't get access to a shower mid-afternoon. After work you're too hungry to work out, but then after dinner you're too full and tired. You don't want to go out in the dark all alone.

Look here... If you are looking for an excuse you will always find one. But if you are looking for a way to get it done, you can always find that instead.

Don't try to squeeze in a workout. Decide in advance for the week, for the month, for the year. Write it down on the calendar. Schedule everything else around it. Schedule your meals and your snacks so that you have just the right nutrition and stomach content for your activity. Exercise Intentionally.

Make sure you schedule plenty of sleep. Go to bed about 9 hours before you plan to exercise. Sleep about 8 hours. You don't want to be up late and trying to exercise without the appropriate sleep.

Google Calendar:

I ♥ Google Calendar. This online tool gives you access to your schedule from any computer or even your smart phone. I enter in everything; all my workouts, where, when, and what I'm doing. Nowadays I do a lot of triathlon training, so it's hard to keep track of all the different activities. Google Calendar helps me keep them all straight.

Even if you are just walking in the evenings, put it on the calendar. Work everything else around it. You said this was a priority in your life. Act like it.

For me, the best feature of Google Calendar is the text message reminders. At 7:00 this morning I woke up to a text message from Google. It said: "Reminder: Run @ Sunday 7:30am". I didn't even have to think about it. The calendar said run, so I ran. It's that simple.

A little scheduling and planning goes a long way. Scheduling is the difference between "best intentions" and your actual behavior. Don't just intend on eating healthy and exercising. Put it on the calendar, schedule around it, and do it.

Chapter 5 - Logging

No this chapter is not about how to become a lumberjack.

It is very important to start logging and tracking everything. Everything? Well... Everything that matters for reaching your goals.

You've set a goal. You need to measure the progress toward your goal. You also need to track, measure, and log all the factors and actions necessary to reach your goal.

Law #5 -
You Can't Manage What You Don't Measure.

Let's take a look at some of the goals we talked about in the last chapter and discuss how we should track, measure, and log for each.

Goal: Get my body fat down to 18% by December 25th.

> Log everything you consume.
>> Know your calorie intake, how much fat, carbs, and protein you consume. Know how much of each nutrient you should consume each day and if you are on target for the day.
>
> Log all of your exercise and training.
>> Log all of your training sessions. How far did you run, how fast, average heart rate. Did you lift weights? Upper or Lower body? How many laps did you swim? How long did it take?
>
> Track your progress toward your goal.
>> What are your measurements and weight? Track it weekly. Are you gradually moving toward your goal?

You see where I'm going with this, right? If you want to be successful at reaching your goal, you're going to need to track your progress and your efforts.

I'm trying to get lean and strong and fast. I use the smart phone application and web page http://www.MyFitnessPal.com to track everything I consume. Every day and every meal, I track exactly what I eat and drink. I use the app to count my calories and the balance of my macronutrients to make sure I have the perfect balance of carbohydrates, fats, and protein.

Also, I use a composition notebook to log all of my exercise. I track how many miles I swim, bike or run, average heart rate, duration of exercise, effort level, how I feel, etc. I track my weight, my measurements, my resting heart rate, everything related to my goals.

What do <u>you</u> need to track? Everything you care about related to your goals. If you want to lose weight, track what you eat, what you burn, what you weigh, etc. If you want to get strong, track your progress in lifting weights. What you track is up to you.

Goal: Do a 5K run / walk next month.

>Track your walking and running activity
>>How often are you walking or running?
>>What distance and duration?
>>How do you feel before during and after?
>>What was your heart rate like during the activity?

Goal: Raise my LBM to 120 lbs by New Year's Day

>Track your body building activities.
>>How often did you do Brazil Butt Lift or P90X?
>>Log your trips to the gym.
>>Track your strength improvements.
>>Measure your Lean Body Mass to monitor the progress.
>>Track your protein intake.

Goal: Drop my resting heart rate to 62 BPM by July 4th.

>Monitor your interval training
>>How often did you do interval training?
>>What was the quality of the training?
>>What heart rate zones did you work in?
>>What are the duration and frequency of your intervals?
>>Monitor your resting heart rate.

These numbers are the key to your success. You have to know what progress looks like. You have to know for sure that you are really working toward your goal.

Why? What is the benefit of all this logging?

First of all, we sometimes think we are doing better or being stricter than we actually are. For example, perhaps you think you ate 1800 calories per day, but you can't lose a pound. You probably really ate 2800 calories instead. Or maybe you only ate 1100 calories and did more harm to your metabolism than good. Don't use guess work.

By knowing exactly what you are doing to reach your goal and the progress toward that goal, you can judge if what you are doing is working and how well.

If you plan to lose 2 pounds per week, but you are typically losing 1.68 pounds per week, you might need to change your routine or change your goal.

Ahhhh, that's right. You can change your goal. That is not failing, that is re-adjusting. If you started off planning to lose 7 pounds per week and now have come to realize that is impossible, change your goal. Push it back three months. Who cares?

Logging allows you to hold yourself accountable. Sure it is a pain in the butt to enter everything you eat, but that is part of the point. I don't want that Nacho Supreme in my log, so I'm not going to eat it. I don't want another blank page in my exercise log, so I'm not going to skip it.

Measure it! Track it! Log it!

Chapter 6 - Why Do We Eat?

Did you say, "Because we get hungry"?   BZZZZ! Wrong!

We eat because our brain sends us chemical signals to eat. Think about it. How many times have you been sitting on the couch watching TV after dinner and suddenly you think, "You know, I could really go for some chocolate"?

You literally just ate dinner. There is no way you are hungry. Why in the world do you want chocolate?

Your brain is this crazy thing that works using all kinds of chemical signals and receptors. When you send your brain the wrong messages by eating the wrong stuff, it returns the favor by sending your stomach the wrong message in return.

Law #6 -
Will power alone cannot overcome your desire to eat.

You can't wish it away. You can't "Just be strong". You can't fight your brain with logic or reason or will power. Your brain is in charge and what it says goes.

Hopeless? Not to me, because I know the secret. If you send your brain the right messages, it will play nice. By eating healthily, your brain gets completely reprogrammed and starts sending your body all the right messages.

Think of the dog chasing his tail. Running in circles over and over again, never catching that darn tail. That's your diet, an endless feedback loop of you fighting with your brain. Break the cycle. Send your brain the right message and it will allow you to live a healthy life. No struggling with your diet and cravings; it will be perfectly natural. You and your brain chemicals working together in harmony.

Sounds great, eh? I bet you are wondering how exactly you do that!

You do that by reading the section and mini-chapters on diet, and then apply it to your life. You do that by following my diet – The Magic Formula.

Let's take a look at some of the chemicals we produce and how they affect you and your diet. In my humble opinion, these are the top 4 chemical contributors causing fake hunger.

Serotonin: Or 5-HT is a monoamine neurotransmitter. It is a large contributor to "feeling of well-being and happiness". It has various functions including regulation of mood, appetite, and sleep, as well as cognitive functions such as memory and learning.

Dopamine: An organic chemical functioning as a neurotransmitter in the brain. It plays a huge role in reward-motivated behavior. Each reward increases the dopamine levels in the brain. Drugs such as cocaine and amphetamines act by amplifying the effects of dopamine, thus the name "dope"

All right I'll admit it. I'm an addict! I crave... I have an uncontrolled yearning for Serotonin and Dopamine. I'd bet you do too!

People who are fighting depression feel down, tired, hopeless. They sometimes lack the will to get out of bed or the desire to live. Why? These two brain chemicals are major contributors.

Serotonin and Dopamine make you feel good. Scratch that. Make you feel great! I can't get enough of the stuff. I sometimes think that my entire life, my entire existence on this planet is boiled down to the search for these two chemicals.

You are supposed to produce these two naturally in well regulated quantities. However some people do not. Those people are doomed to a miserable existence unless they find a way to increase their levels. Most try to do it through drugs like anti-depressants or recreational narcotics and alcohol. But I would offer an alternative. Exercise and diet.

Serotonin and Dopamine are reward-driven; produced whenever your behavior meets the requirement. What kind of behavior works?

- Over Eating: When you eat, particularly when you gorge, your brain unloads Serotonin. This causes you to crave food even when you're not hungry. You do not want food. You are just looking for your next fix. You're a junkie and your drug of choice is food.

- Sex: When done correctly, this activity releases huge amounts of Dopamine and Serotonin. During your next orgasm, lean your head back, close your eyes and feel these drugs release into your brain. The euphoric feeling of these brain chemicals is far more intense and satisfying than anything you'll feel in your genitals.

- Risky Behavior: Sky diving, rocky mountain climbing, going two point seven seconds on a bull named Fu Manchu, these are all high risk behaviors which produce huge chemical responses in your brain. Driving 120MPH, robbing a bank, or BASE jumping are all good for getting your next fix!

- Recreational Drugs: Aside from the cost, the jail time, and the long term effects on the body, recreational drugs are counterproductive to the goal. Users actually produce less and less dopamine naturally, causing you to need more and more drugs. Basically, these diminishing returns do more harm than good.

- Vigorous Exercise: This is my favorite. I try to avoid over eating. Sex is a couple's activity. Risky behavior is... well... risky. Which leaves vigorous exercise. When you exercise you get an intense brain chemical release. The longer and harder the exercise, the more fulfilling the reward. It is amazing how you hurt and ache and can't breathe, feeling like you're about to die, yet the brain chemical reward is so intense that you feel great. You feel awful, but you feel great.

Cortisol: Also known as hydrocortisone, a steroid hormone produced in the adrenal cortex. Released in response to stress and a low level of blood glucocorticoids. Its primary functions are to increase blood sugar and suppress the immune system.

Cortisol is considered the stress hormone. When you have bad stress in your life, your adrenal gland overproduces cortisol. After years of being overworked and over stressed you can develop Adrenal Fatigue. Cortisol, like insulin, is instrumental for blood sugar production and absorption. So, if you screw up your adrenal function, you screw up your ability to deal with carbohydrates (sugar).

Bottom line concerning cortisol; too much stress in your life, along with a bad diet causes your hormones to get all wackadoodle (that's a technical term). That makes you have a desire to eat inappropriate amounts of food at inappropriate times of the day.

Insulin: A peptide hormone produced in the pancreas, is central in fat and sugar metabolism.

When you eat carbohydrates (sugar) they go through your stomach and then straight into your blood stream. Your body has this magic chemical for processing (metabolizing) that blood sugar and turning it into energy (stored glycogen and or eventually ATP) called insulin. This hormone converts your food to energy. The glycogen gets stored in your muscles and the ATP is burned up for work.

If you overwhelm your body with too many carbs, your pancreas can't produce enough insulin to keep up. After years of poor eating habits you can develop Metabolic Syndrome. This can lead to Insulin Resistance and eventually you develop Diabetes.

At this point your pancreas is damaged from years of abuse and now you have to take hormone supplement injections several times a day for the rest of your life. Nice job.

I digress. Now that you know how insulin works, what does it have to do with making you feel hungry? Awesome question, I'm glad you asked.

When you eat carbohydrates and dump sugar into your blood causing a blood sugar spike, your pancreas kicks into high gear producing insulin. Soon thereafter the insulin eats up all the sugar. The pancreas doesn't instantly turn off when the sugar is gone. It has a bit of a delayed reaction and continues to dump insulin into your blood. Next thing you know, these chemicals cause you to start craving food again.

Let's say you have a nice sour dough bagel for breakfast. (spike) Two hours later you're ready for second breakfast (crash), so you grab a doughnut. (spike) A little while later you are ready for lunch. (crash) You grab some soft tacos and finally feel satiated. (spike) Next thing you know you're falling asleep at your desk. (crash). It's what I call the Insulin Rollercoaster, and it will cause diabetes!

Law #7 -
The Insulin Rollercoaster, nobody rides for free!

Easy solution, avoid meals with a high glycemic load. I did not say avoid carbs. Manage carbs.

Read your nutritional information on restaurant web sites. Read the labels on food. Enter it into MyFitnessPal app to read the nutritional content. Make sure that the net carbs (total carbs minus fiber) are not too high. The sugar shouldn't be too high relative to the fiber, fat, and protein. If there is too much carbohydrate, then you get a high glycemic load and you will have problems.

Water: Your body is about 50% to 70% water. We drink water for hydration and for electrolytes which are essential for neurological functions such as muscle control, breathing, heart beating, thinking, etc. Additionally, it's required for flushing foods and toxins out of your system. Chances are you are not drinking enough water.

So what, you ask? Most people cannot distinguish thirst from hunger. Yeah, yeah, yeah; you can obviously tell the difference between a dry mouth and a growling from the pit of your abdomen. But often you are not hungry, you are just craving something. You stand in front of the refrigerator or pantry trying to figure out what you are craving. It is water! Drink it!

Nutrients: Your body requires certain micronutrients to function properly. Vitamins and minerals, iron, calcium, potassium, antioxidants, essential fatty acids, and countless other nutrients are required for healthy living.

When you lack these nutrients in your diet, your body will crave these nutrients. You must eat a healthy diet with all the required micronutrients or else you will have a hard time feeling satiated.

Back to the question. Why do we eat?

If we have a healthy lifestyle with the appropriate diet and exercise. We eat in order to replenish the requisite nutrients. If you are not controlling your body chemistry through proper diet and exercise, you eat because your chemistry is out of control.

Law #8 -
You must control your body chemistry to control your appetite.

Are you hungry or do you just think you're hungry?

Is your craving really for food or are you just thirsty?

Do you want to eat or do you just want to feel better by secreting serotonin and dopamine?

Is it time for a meal or are you just riding the Insulin Rollercoaster?

Before I learned about this topic I really did not understand what hunger felt like. I honestly could not even tell if I was hungry or not. I thought I was hungry all of the time. I learned hunger should not be experienced in your head, but in the pit of your stomach. Learn the difference.

One last note: Next time you accuse one of your skinny friends of "having a good metabolism", you might want to consider instead that they just have good body and brain chemistry. You can have that too. It's not genetic, it's intentional.

(Ok, maybe it's a little genetic, but that wouldn't be nearly as dramatic of an ending to this chapter)

Chapter 7 - Metabolism

Everybody who is overweight, my former self included, likes to think they have a slow metabolism. "I can't lose any weight because my metabolism is too slow." I've heard it, I've said it, I've lived it. The truth is, with the exception of certain medical conditions, you are in complete control over your own metabolism.

Your body is responding to your actions by altering its chemistry. It's like your body is a computer and you are a computer programmer. Your computer is just going to run whatever code you upload into it. If you're loading bad code, you're going to crash your computer. Ain't nobody got time for that. (BTW, if you're not laughing at that expression, you need to watch the video. Google it.)

It is up to you to program your body correctly by eating the right food at the right time and getting appropriate exercise and rest. Doing so will kick your metabolism into overdrive.

Law #9 -
You are in complete control of your metabolism.

Let's take a look at the contemporary classic analogy; your metabolism is like a campfire.

Your body is actually very similar to a campfire. Both require that you add a quality fuel source to burn, wood for the fire and food for your body. They both burn all day and night to produce energy. The campfire produces heat energy to keep you warm, while your metabolism provides energy to perform. They both need to be nurtured to burn well.

Breakfast is called "breakfast" because you were fasting all night. Now that you are awake you can break your fast by eating break-fast. Get it? Eating breakfast is like lighting the campfire, the flame has gone out and it is time to light the fire and get things burning again.

Your body is sitting there stagnant waiting for you to flip the switch and turn it back on for the day. It is waiting for you to send it the message that it is time to turn on your metabolism and start burning fuel.

Are you one of those people who do not eat breakfast? Maybe you're always in a hurry in the morning. Maybe it gives you a little tummy-ache. I completely understand. But here's the bad news for you... You are going to have to get over it because you are doomed to poor health until you start eating a healthy breakfast each and every day. Sorry.

As for the tummy-ache, it goes away. If you don't often eat breakfast you will probably have a tough time making the transition to a breakfast person. But after a few weeks it will feel perfectly natural with no problems. I promise.

Incidentally, author Mark Hyman, M.D. likes to refer to skipping breakfast as a big part of the "Sumo Wrestler Diet" because it can really help you pack on the pounds.

Law #10 - Breakfast really is the most important meal of the day.

Back to the campfire. If you've ever been camping, you know it is not easy to build a good campfire. There is always somebody that wants to throw a bunch of wood in a pile and try to light it. But that won't work. In order to build a good campfire you really need to do it right.

You start off with a clean empty fire pit and a nice pile of wood. You plan out the fire by gathering various piles of wood of varying sizes. You start off with some small kindling for the base layer of the campfire. Next you add some small twigs, followed by small branches. As you light the campfire the kindling burns up quickly, but does a nice job of igniting the small branches. Now you can throw on larger and larger branches and logs until finally you have a nice blazing campfire.

But you can't just walk away from it and expect it to keep burning. You need to tend your campfire, constantly adding fuel. You must feed your fire the right fuel at the right time in order to keep it burning.

If you want to have a good healthy metabolism burning all day, you need to treat your metabolism like a campfire. Start off with the right breakfast to get your fire started. Then give your body good quality fuel in small doses every few hours. That means small well balanced meals with low glycemic load every three to four hours.

If you skip breakfast in the morning, eat lunch at noon, eat dinner 8 hours later, then a late night snack at midnight, don't complain about your slow metabolism.

Law #11 -
Eat a healthy snack or meal every 3 to 4 hours.

Calories, Weight Loss and Your Metabolism

There are several schools of thought on the best way to lose weight. You have your Dieters, you have your Weight Lifters and you have your Runners. Let's see who has it right.

It is commonly believed that a pound of fat contains 3500 calories. Meaning, in order to lose one pound of fat you need a deficiency of 3500 calories. Or, if you eat 3500 calories more than you burn, you will gain one pound of fat.

So if you want to lose 100 pounds all you have to do is burn 350,000 calories. Running for two straight months non-stop will do nicely. I bet there is a better alternative.

But before we can get too deep into this subject, we need to understand Basal Metabolic Rate (BMR).

Metabolism

BMR

Your Basal Metabolic Rate is essentially the number of calories (the amount of energy) you consume just existing. There are lots of factors that go into your BMR, including:

- Resting Heart Rate
- Lean Body Mass
- Total Fat Mass
- Body Temperature
- Age
- Climate
- Brain activity and function
- Illness
- Fitness level
- Typical activity level

Your BMR makes up the vast majority of calories burned per day. People are always looking toward exercise to burn extra calories, but the truth is that your daily activity typically accounts for about 20% of your daily calorie burn.

The following chart shows that depending on your activity level, BMR makes up approximately 70% of your total calorie consumption, while activity and digestion consume the rest.

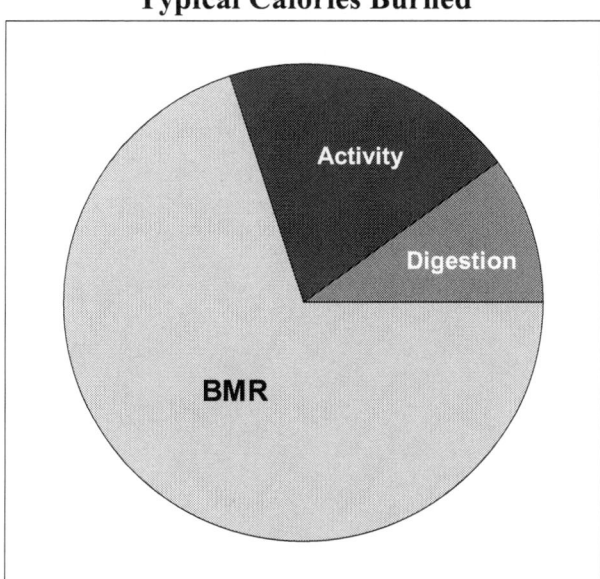

Typical Calories Burned

Your body is basically one big space heater, burning up calories producing heat, regulating body temperature, brain and organ function, etc. It's rumored that Olympic gold medalist swimmer Michael Phelps burns 12,000 calories per day. This is due to body temperature regulation. He literally burns thousands of calories heating his swimming pool with his own body.

Take a look at a breakdown of your BMR to see where all those calories are going.

BMR Break Down Chart

*BMR and body weight in men (Harris & Benedict, 1919)

Every body is different. Some people have a really high BMR, while others are really low. The following chart shows the wide variation in measured BMR based on the Harris & Benedict Study.

Calorie Burn vs. Body Weight Kg

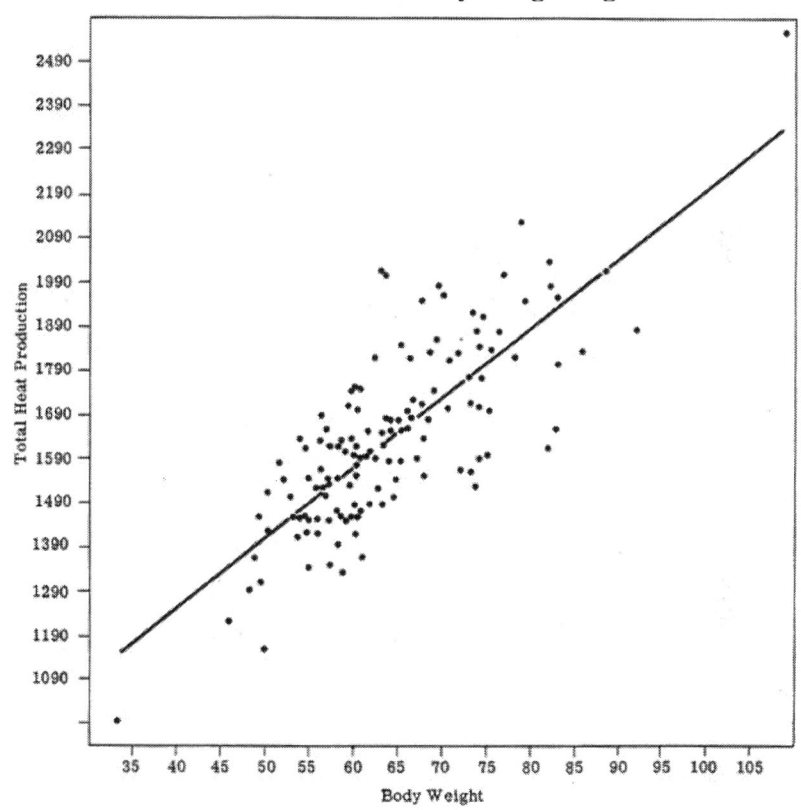

BMR and body weight in men (Harris & Benedict, 1919)

As you can see in the chart above, there is a wide variation in BMR from individual to individual.

In the light of your new understanding of Basal Metabolic Rate, let's get back to our discussion of Dieters, Weight Lifters, and Runners.

Dieters

The basic mindset of your typical dieter is "If I consume fewer calories I will lose weight." This is true for all intents and purposes. However, there are tons of problems with this Thermodynamic Approach to weight loss.

Before we get into the problems, let's look at how dieting works. The main concept here is that a pound of fat consists of 3500 calories. Therefore, you can lose one pound of fat for every 3500 calories of deficiency.

If you want to lose one pound per week, 3500 calories over 7 days is 500 calories per day. If your BMR is 1800 calories per day, your food limit is only 1300 calories per day.

If you want to lose two pounds per week, 7000 calories over 7 days is 1000 calories per day. If your BMR is 1800 calories per day, your food limit is only 800 calories per day.

I think you can probably see the problem already. How the heck are you supposed to function on 800 calories per day? You'll get sick. You'll be tired, no energy, dark circles under your eyes. If you want to lose 50 pounds, do you really want to eat 800 calories per day for 6 months?!

How in the world are you going to keep a healthy metabolism eating only 800 to 1300 calories per day? You're not!

To the contrary, your body is going to fight back. Your metabolism is going to think there is a food shortage, the beginning of another ice age. Now your body will shift into starvation mode, trying to conserve every ounce of fat stored on your body for the coming nuclear winter.

Law #12 -
Your body will cling to fat when in starvation mode.

Here's the cliché, get ready for it... You gotta eat to lose!

But really, it's true. You must consume plenty of food or your body will start to shut down. The longer you diet, the lower your Basal Metabolic Rate. After years of yoyo dieting, your BMR will drop so low that everything you eat becomes body fat.

Metabolism

If you've been dieting for years, you must let your metabolism recover if you want to have any hope of losing weight.

Speaking of losing weight... You should have no interest in just "losing weight". Your concern should be losing fat. Which brings us to the second major problem with dieting. When you diet having a daily calorie deficiency, your body must consume itself, literally burning human flesh to produce energy for brain and organ function.

Unfortunately for you, your metabolism does not discriminate too much as to what it decides to burn up. When losing weight from dieting, you are eating up your fat AND your muscle. If you are not careful about your methods, you'll lose just as much muscle as fat. This is bad.

Law #13 -
Dieting will eat up your muscles.

It sounds a little like dieting is a hopeless way to lose weight, but that's not true either. Actually, dieting may be the best way to lose weight if managed correctly. But it is very tricky to do it well. Let's make up a few rules for successful dieting.

- Losing one or two pounds per week is the limit. Never plan to lose any more than that.

- You must fight off starvation mode. Keep the campfire burning.

- You must keep your daily calorie deficiency small. Don't go in to calorie debt by more than 500 calories under your BMR.

- Burn extra calories with aerobic exercise.

- Fight to keep your muscles with weight training.

- Have weekly Metabolic Recovery Days when you consume a large quantity of healthy calories.

- Use a diet that mimics the diet you want to eat permanently for your new healthy lifestyle.

Weight Lifters

The second school of thought among these "losers" are the weight lifters. If you recall from the graphical break down of BMR, one of the big components of BMR is Skeletal Muscle. Let me break it down for you...

The more muscle mass you have, the more calories you burn sitting on the couch. The weight lifters ask, why would you deprive yourself 500 calories per day when you could simply build a little extra muscle mass and burn those calories during the night while you sleep?

The Sterling-Pasmore Equation says that your BMR = LBM x 13.8

Think about it; for every pound of muscle you add on, you can afford to eat another 13.8 calories. That doesn't sound like much, but 10 pounds of muscle is an extra serving of lean protein.

My LBM is currently 167 pounds; therefore my BMR is 2305 calories per day.

Law #14 -
Muscle Mass burns calories.

How about we do some weight training to burn calories, increase our BMR and improve our muscle tone to get a lean sexy body?

If you are a woman and you are worried about gaining too much muscle, don't fret over it. The only way you are going to look too muscular is if you get your body fat down below 10% or start taking testosterone supplements. (Don't get any ideas fellas!)

Runners

The last group of "big fat losers" are the runners. Well, they're not all runners. Actually, we are talking about anybody who's keen on weight loss through aerobic exercise.

The main principle they subscribe to is: to earn a caloric deficiency not through diet, not through high BMR, but though burning calories during aerobic exercise. These people ask, why would anybody diet when you could just go for a run?

To do this effectively, you need to get your heart rate up and keep it there. We'll talk about heart rate zone training later.

How much weight can be lost during exercise? A lot. You can use a smart phone app like MyFitnessPal, NikePlus, or MapMyRide to automatically calculate the calories burned. I prefer to get a heart rate monitor and a stop watch, using the following equation[1].

Cal = Calories
A = Age
W = Weight
HR = Heart Rate
T = Time in Minutes

Men:
$$Cal = \frac{[(A \times 0.2017) + (W \times 0.09036) + (HR \times 0.6309) - 55.0969] \times T}{4.184}$$

Women:
$$Cal = \frac{[(A \times 0.074) + (W \times 0.05741) + (HR \times 0.4472) - 20.4022] \times T}{4.184}$$

If that's too much for you, just use an on-line calculator like I do.

Or use the built into the TWB Smart Digital Scale, available on Amazon.com

---

[1] *Keytel LR, Goedecke JH, Noakes TD, Hiiloskorpi H, Laukkanen R, van der Merwe L, Lambert EV. Prediction of energy expenditure from heart rate monitoring during submaximal exercise. J Sports Sci. 2005 Mar;23(3):289-97.*

So how does this all add up? Let's say you are a 42 year old woman weighing 175 pounds.

Activity	Duration	Avg HR	Calories
Walking	60 Minutes	125	698
Running	45 Minutes	163	706
Biking	120 Minutes	142	1613
Racquetball	50 Minutes	185	902
Beach Body Insanity	42 Minutes	173	704
Swimming	39 Minutes	129	470

Doing a little exercise goes a long way. As you can see, one aerobic exercise session can really help you build your calorie deficit.

Should you start a regular aerobic exercise routine? Heck Yeah!

Back to the question… Who's right, the Dieters, the Weight Lifters, or the Runners? Well of course, they are all right. In order to lose fat and boost your metabolism you really need all three methods.

A healthy lifestyle isn't just one of these methods. You must eat a healthy diet. You must have a healthy Lean Body Mass. You must get off your butt and do a little exercise. All three of these in combination will give you the best results.

However, it really does depend on your own personal goals. Use these three methods in the right combination to achieve your personal fitness goals.

Warning: Exercise may make you eat or drink more calories than you burn. If you are rewarding yourself with a BigMac just because you ran a few miles, you are doing more harm than good.

The fact is, when you exercise vigorously you really need more calories and food. Just be careful to do the math right and not be self-defeating. Doing the cardio work is very often self-defeating because on cardio days you eat more and generally do less activity (because you're tired).

My recommendation... If you're trying to lose a bunch of weight, lay off the high intensity cardio for a while. Do cardio, but stay in Heart Rate Zones 1 and 2. We'll talk more about that later.

If you're going to do intense cardio training, you'll need to be very careful to keep your appetite under control.

Thermogenics and Negative Calorie Foods

You can see in the pie chart that your daily calorie burn comes from three different areas; BMR, Activity, and Digestion. It's true, digesting the food you eat consumes a lot of calories, somewhere around 8% of your daily burn. You can actually increase the number of calories burned in digestion with thermogenics and negative calorie foods.

Semantically speaking, there is no such thing as a negative calorie food. All food contains some chemical energy and therefore always has some calories. However, if a food takes more calories to digest than it provides, it is considered a negative calorie food.

The classic example is raw celery stalks, which are thought to take more calories to digest than are consumed. We are not talking about cooked celery, or celery with peanut butter, or celery with vegetable dip, just plain old raw celery all by itself.

Now for the sad news... There really is not a lot of scientific evidence to back up the claim that celery (or any other food) takes more calories to digest than it contains. Despite the fact that there may be no truly negative calorie foods, the idea still holds true; some foods require more digestive energy. There are many foods which are very low in calories which make the list.

Bottom line, whether or not they are truly negative calorie foods does not matter too much to me. These foods make a quick and healthy snack that you grab without worrying about adding to your bottom line.

- Apples
- Cranberries
- Grapefruit
- Lemon
- Mango
- Orange
- Garlic
- Pineapple
- Raspberries
- Strawberries
- Tangerine
- Onion
- Green Beans
- Radishes
- Asparagus
- Beets
- Broccoli
- Cabbage
- Cauliflower
- Celery
- Spinach
- Peppers
- Cucumber
- Dandelion
- Endive
- Garden Cress
- Lettuce
- Turnips

Again, "negative calorie food" is half urban legend and half-truth. The whole truth is these are good wholesome foods with very low calories and high nutrition.

Thermogenics are stimulant foods that tend to produce heat in the body during digestion and metabolism. These thermogenics will tend to increase your BMR as well. While there are plenty of healthy natural thermogenic foods to choose from, caffeine and ephedrine are unhealthy thermogenics,

All of the negative calorie foods listed above are considered thermogenics. Additionally, green tea, ginger, alpha lipoic acid, hot peppers and spices, coconut oil, apple cider vinegar, grapefruit, and ice water all have significant thermogenic effects.

Chapter 8 - Ice Age Metabolism

Whether you think we evolved or we were created, one thing is for sure, our bodies were made for a different time. During most of the history of mankind, life was hard. Our days were spent hunting and gathering.

For most of history, life was a struggle. Every day was a search for resources just to stay alive. Even in modern history, most people spent all day tending their crops and animals, raising barns, and working hard. There were no desk jobs, there were no televisions, grocery stores, or microwave ovens. If you wanted to eat some food you either had to find it, kill it, or grow it. Times certainly have changed.

Your body is a finely tuned machine capable of amazing things. The body chemistry alone is a wonderful symphony of chemical signals and receptors, all working together to send messages to the body and brain. These chemical messages are the feedback mechanism so your body can adjust for any situation at hand, including an ice age.

During an ice age, you have very limited food resources and very high work load. When you restrict calories and work hard, your body notices and triggers starvation mode. This brings the metabolism to a screeching halt. Your body tries its hardest to conserve every ounce of fat and hold on to every calorie.

This is a critical survival mechanism for the entire human race. If you're fat, you should be happy knowing you'd do very well in the next climate crisis.

The Modern Ice Age

Unfortunately, our bodies have not had time to adjust to this new period in history, a time of excess. The easy life of watching TV, working at a desk, and eating heavily processed foods is too much for our bodies to handle. Next thing you know, you start packing on the pounds.

After we've gained 15, 20, 25 pounds we all react the same way, by going on a diet and starting to exercise more. That is when we start our own personal modern ice age metabolism.

Think about Law #12 – Your body will cling to fat while in starvation mode. Which brings us to one of the most common myths in the world of diet and exercise: "If I just eat less and exercise more, I will lose weight." Don't believe it!

Why Eat Less - Exercise More does not work.

Are you sending your body the right message? When you go on a calorie restrictive diet and start an exercise program, you are sending your body two very specific messages.

1. Hey there body… Look out, there is a food shortage.

2. And by the way, hard times have arrived. Expect to do some extra work.

What happens when you send these two messages to the body? It thinks winter has come and starts to react to the signals you are giving it. It literally starts to lower your Basal Metabolic Rate, lower and lower with each passing day of diet and exercise.

After months or years of this activity of yoyo dieting, your body can't handle any more of it. Every time you go on a diet you lose a few pounds, but gain back even more. That is because once you go back to your "normal" diet with your crippled metabolism you can't help but gain weight.

Law #15 -
Simply Eating Less & Exercising More does not work.

The problem is that you are sending your body the wrong messages. Packing on the pounds is the exact correct response to the signals you are sending to your body. Remember what I said earlier, you are in complete control over your metabolism. Your skinny friends don't have better genes, they have better chemistry.

That's why a fat guy like me can diet and train vigorously for triathlon all year and never shed a single pound off my total body mass.

How do you rev up your metabolism? How do you avoid your ice age metabolism? By sending your body the right message. Instead of telling your body there is a food shortage and hard work is expected, you want to give it messages that will allow it to shed fat.

1. There is plenty of food. No need to store fat.
2. Life is easy, I'm not expecting too much from you.

Basically, I'm saying Eat More, Exercise Less!

But, but, but... That's what made me fat?! How am I supposed to lose fat by doing the same thing that made me fat?

It is a difficult balancing act. You want to restrict calories through diet and burn extra calories through exercise, but do it without your body noticing and reacting.

What the heck! How do you do that?

Therein lies the rub. The trick is to:

- Restrict your calories, but not too much. Your deficit should be only a few hundred calories per day, maybe 500 calories max.
- Exercise, but not too much. You want to stick to heart rate zone one. Actually, walking an hour a day is probably the single best exercise for fat loss. Swimming, water aerobics, and cycling are all very effective too.
- Have Metabolic Recovery Days once per week when you consume a much higher number of calories. This is not a "cheat day". You are not cheating if it is part of the diet. And that doesn't mean go eat a pizza and 6 hotdogs. You should continue to eat the right foods, just a lot more of them.

Law #16 -
To lose weight, you must send your body the right messages.

Excessive high intensity training along with a calorie restrictive diet is certainly counterproductive to your weight loss goals. You gotta eat to lose.

Chapter 9 - Lifestyle Change

Quoting my very favorite economist, "When you want to help people, you tell them the truth. When you want to help yourself, you tell them what they want to hear." - *Thomas Sowell*

What most people want to hear is that this is easy; there is some magic bullet out there that will make you lose fat, gain muscle and live a healthy life. The painful truth is that this is difficult. It is a complex puzzle that you must solve for yourself.

You can't just go on a diet, lose a bunch of weight, and then go back to business as usual. It does not work that way. It takes a serious lifestyle change and a commitment to your new lifestyle. You can't have one foot in and one foot out of a healthy lifestyle. You must commit to it.

Have you ever been on a diet and had this happen?

You see somebody eating something you are forbidden to eat. You think to yourself, "I can't have that because I'm on a diet." But then you realize you have a cheat day coming soon. "I can't eat that today because I'm on a diet. But come Sunday I'm getting my cheat day and I'm going to eat those Oreo cookies."

If you've had those thoughts you are not committed to your new healthy lifestyle. Let's say you were addicted to crack, you can't have crack on your cheat days. If something is a poisonous toxin and not fit for human consumption, you must expel it from your life permanently and forever. Not just while you are on the diet, not just until your next cheat day, forever.

Lifestyle change is not temporary. It is a permanent commitment to spending the rest of your life eating healthy and getting appropriate exercise. Are you ready to make that commitment to yourself and the people who love you?

Law #17 -
Permanent weight loss requires a permanent lifestyle change.

Do Diets Work?

80% - 95% of dieters fail to have sustained weight loss. There are some studies showing with certain group diet programs only two in a thousand people keep off their weight for 5 years or more.

Why do the vast majority of dieters fail? Because the diet is temporary. If you want to be successful at permanent weight loss and a healthy life, you must make permanent changes to your lifestyle.

Don't Go on a diet	**Do** Find a healthy diet you can live with for life
Don't Work off extra pounds	**Do** Find an exercise plan for life
Don't Eat crap food on cheat days	**Do** Decide which foods you are willing to put in your body and which foods you are not

I can't tell you what you want to hear. I must tell you the truth. You must be willing to make a long term commitment to a healthy lifestyle in order to be successful. Accept that you must behave a certain way in order to get the results you are looking for. A permanent lifestyle change is in order.

The Good News

Once you start down this road it actually becomes addictive. Eating good nutritious food makes you feel great and eating crappy food makes you feel crappy. Once you figure that out, you'll want to stick to your new healthy diet.

When everybody else is eating birthday cake by the pound, you won't skip it because "you're on a diet". You will sample a little, but once you taste it you'll realize that a big plate of highly processed carbohydrates will make you feel like crap. After eating healthy whole foods for a year or so, you'll see those types of processed foods as disgusting, even toxic.

The exercise is even more addictive. Once you start dosing yourself with a rush of brain chemicals produced during exercise, you'll want more and more.

Chapter 10 - Water, Water Everywhere

Drinking a lot of water is critically important for living a healthy life. Not just for dieting, but as part of your normal everyday diet and as part of all your exercise activities.

You might say something like: "I drink plenty of water. I get water in my coffee, in my iced tea, and in my soda. Everything I drink has water in it." Sorry, you know that answer is B.S.!

There are lots and lots of benefits to drinking water, ranging from heart health all the way to good brain function. Skipping the water and drinking some alternative simply will not give you the same health benefits. Drink water, not tea, not juice, not Vitamin Water, just plain old water.

Soda and Diet Soda

Soda may be the absolute worst American dietary staple! I can't think of anything less appealing to a healthy diet. You take perfectly good water and then saturate it with 17 teaspoons of High Fructose Corn Syrup (HFCS). Nothing like drinking 120 empty calories of highly processed, laboratory made carbohydrates.

DON'T DRINK IT! STOP! It is toxic and it is killing you, literally. Diabetes kills about a quarter million Americans per year, plus causes blindness in approximately four million Americans per year. High sugar diets are also a leading contributor to heart disease, the number one killer in America! Quit drinking soda!

I like to think of soda as dessert. I could have a slice of cake or a nice cold orange soda. Same thing from a nutritional perspective.

What about diet soda? Sure, it has no calories and no HFCS, but what takes the place? Toxic Artificial Sweeteners! Ask yourself, do I really want to be drinking a laboratory chemical, developed by accident, thrown into drinks just because it happens to taste sweet? I've heard cyanide taste like almonds; would you put that in your brownie mix? No, because it will kill you immediately.

In my opinion, based on everything I've read, artificial sweeteners are poisonous toxins not fit for human consumption. They will make you sick, cause cancer, and generally hurt your health and longevity. Our government seems to think these products are just dandy based on studies done by the chemical companies producing the products. All I can say to them is, SHAME ON YOU! Lobbyist and campaign funds must be more important than public safety.

But hey, that's just my opinion.

(By the way, I had to say it's only my opinion so I don't get sued)

Milk

I'm sure you've heard of Lactose, one of the main nutrients in milk. Lactose, like anything ending in "ose" is sugar. (e.g. lactose, fructose, and glucose) Basically, drinking a glass of milk is the equivalent of drinking a glass of sugar. *Don't worry, it has a bunch of fat too.*

150 calories, 13 grams of sugar, 8 grams of fat, does not sound very healthy to me. Don't even get me started on the hormones and antibiotics they pump into the cows.

Milk does have some redeeming qualities, so I shouldn't be quite so hard on it. It does have a nice quantity of the protein casein. Plus it has added vitamin D, calcium and other vitamins. But to me, the good aspects certainly do not outweigh the bad.

Juice

Many people think of juice as a healthy alternative to soda because it is natural. First of all, you'd really need to put in a serious effort to find an all-natural juice product. Most of the products on the market are highly processed, filled with extra sugar and preservatives.

Even if you are making your own organic juice from your very own garden, it's still not a really healthy choice. When you take fruit and strip out the fiber, you are left with a high sugar, high glycemic index beverage. I can hear the insulin roller coaster rolling in.

Law #18 -
Don't Drink Calories! Avoid high sugar drinks.

There are lots of drink alternatives. But if you are trying to lose weight, live a healthy life with a healthy diet and exercise, there really is only one drink for you. Water. Drink water. Nothing else, just water.

How much water should you drink?
It seems that everybody has their own opinion about how much water is right for you. The right answer is, "a lot". Some experts say eight to ten 8oz glasses per day, while others say to drink a 1/2 ounce for every pound of body mass.

When you lose fluids through exercise, you will need even more. You need at least 20oz more per hour of exercise.

How can you tell if you're drinking enough water? You spend half the day running to the bathroom. Your urine should be mostly clear, unless you are loading up on B vitamins.

Law #19 -
Drink Water. Drink 1/2 Oz for every pound of body mass.

What are the benefits of water?
Drinking water has lots and lots of benefits, more than I can mention here. But I will go over some of the top benefits as they apply to your healthy journey.

Hydration
I hate to state the obvious, but water keeps you hydrated. Every other drink has lots of extra ingredients which impede hydration. Nothing quenches your body's thirst like water.

Nothing in your body functions correctly unless you are properly hydrated. Brain, heart, kidneys, liver, muscles, everything in your body needs water to function. Drink water to keep your body functioning.

Avoiding false hunger

As I mentioned earlier, sometimes it is hard to distinguish between hunger and thirst. Sometimes you think you are hungry, but really you are thirsty.

You have to stay hydrated to avoid a false sense of hunger.

Keeps your stomach full

Water suppresses your appetite so you don't eat as much. Drinking lots of water means your stomach always has something to process. Pouring in water keeps you from eating too much food. I like to have three 12oz glasses with every meal to help make me feel full.

Neurological function and electrolytes

Normal tap water and bottled water contain electrolytes. Skip the distilled water, it is not made for consumption and has zero electrolytes.

Electrolytes are absolutely critical for brain and neurological function. Potassium, sodium, magnesium, and calcium are all great for you at appropriate levels.

The more you sweat the more electrolytes you lose and need to replenish. I add salt and potassium tablets to my water bottle during long bike rides.

Increases metabolism

Keeping hydrated makes all of your organs work better. In our context that is particularly important for the kidneys and liver. When they get a little dehydrated it impedes your ability to metabolize stored fat and blood sugars.

Flushes toxins from your body

Water is very important for flushing every day toxins out of your body. It's like taking a shower on the inside of your body. When you are burning fat, all those toxins that are stored in your body fat are released. You need to flush them out quickly before they get reattached to your body.

Better digestive and bowel function

Water and good hydration are very important to proper digestive and bowel function. If you are not properly hydrated you will get constipated. Needless to say, that is not good.

When your bowels are functioning correctly, your body can extract the nutrients from your food effectively. Water helps the nutrients move through your digestive system and into your blood stream.

Immune System

Drinking plenty of water helps fight flu and other illness. Perhaps it is the constant hand washing from going to the bathroom all day.

Thermogenic Affect

Drinking ice water raises your BMR. Your body uses lots of calories to bring that cold water up to 98 degrees.

Drink water. Skip the caffeine, skip the sugar, drink water. Drinking lots of water (particularly ice-water) will keep your body running strong.

Diet
Chapter 11 - Eating Intentionally

Let's get back to the question of why we eat. We discussed why most people eat; because they are at war with their own body chemistry which drives them to eat the wrong stuff at the wrong time. But what about once we have our body chemistry under control? When and what should we be eating?

Perhaps your drive to eat comes from hunger, your body telling you it is time to eat. But just because we are hungry does not give us license to eat whatever we want. We need to eat intentionally.

Instead of eating because you are hungry, eat because you want to consume some specific nutrients.

Food is like a Drug. Are you a user or an abuser? What's your prescription?

Decide in advance what nutrients you want in your body. Decide what proportions of macronutrients, micronutrients, vitamins, minerals, fillers and chemicals you want to ingest. How much of each nutrient do you want to consume and when do you want to do it?

Whenever you are eating a meal, think of it as filling a prescription. Think of yourself as a pharmacist filling a prescription. The doctor says you need a certain number of grams of fat, protein, and carbohydrates, now it is up to you to craft a meal that fills the prescription by giving you the right nutrients.

Law #20 -
You must eat intentionally to have a healthy diet & lifestyle.

The natural tendency for people is to simply "try to eat healthy". That means they do their best to make healthy selections. But if you simply try to make "healthy selections", then take a look at your food log, you might find that your nutritional intake was far from optimal.

Perhaps you select healthy fibrous carbohydrates and healthy unsaturated fats, but you still don't get the proportions right. Too much sodium, not enough protein, low in Omega 3 fatty acid, too high in Omega 6. When you eat intentionally as if you are filling a prescription, you start to get all the numbers right and you will get great results.

Let's run through an example.

Intentionally Eating at Chipotle example:

You go into a Chipotle Mexican Grill restaurant to grab a quick lunch. There are plenty of healthy choices there; it should be easy to eat a healthy meal.

You get yourself a nice steak burrito on a flour tortilla, stuffed with white rice, lettuce, tomato, a little cheese and sour cream. Let's toss in a side of chips and salsa. Sounds yummy! And since it is from Chipotle "Food with Integrity", it must be healthy. Right?

Let's analyze those choices and see.

By the way, I am using the Nutritional Calculator on their web page. It's awesome and I applaud Chipotle for their commitment to health.

Your "healthy" meal has:
- 1485 calories
- 65 grams of fat
- 2760 mg sodium
- 161 grams of carbohydrates

Not looking so healthy now, is it? That flour tortilla loaded you up on salt and carbs. The steak, cheese and sour cream were loaded with fat. Those chips were loaded with salt and carbs. And that white rice is going to spike your blood sugar through the roof!

Diet - Eating Intentionally

What happens if instead of eating randomly, you eat intentionally? You would select chicken instead of beef because it has less saturated and total fat. You would certainly skip the rice and the flour tortilla and trade them in for some healthy black beans. Skip the sour cream and trade it in for some healthy guacamole. Leave the corn chips for the next guy.

Now you've dramatically reduced the glycemic load, balanced your macronutrients and converted a not so healthy meal into a delicious and nutritious healthy meal. You've filled your prescription by eating the right combination of nutrients.

- 485 Calories
- 20 grams of fat (only 4 grams saturated fat)
- Under 1000 mg of sodium
- Only 15 grams of net carbs (33g carbs minus 18g fiber)
- 41 grams of protein!

Why go to a restaurant with so many healthy choices if you are just going to make bad selections?

In the next few chapters we will talk about what you want to consume and why. We will discuss the pros and cons of each nutrient to help you find the right prescription for yourself.

I will often use MyFitnessPal to look up the food I'm planning to eat before ordering, just to confirm that the nutritional information matches my prescription. That way I can make the appropriate adjustments before I eat. I make sure in advance that my macronutrients are balanced.

Remember that your body is like a computer and your food is like a computer program. Your body will run whatever program you upload. Eating intentionally loads your computer with the code to live a happy and healthy life.

Chapter 12 - Fact or Fiction

It is truly saddening to see all the health and diet misconceptions floating around out there. Obesity in America is climbing at alarming rates and it seems that people really don't understand why.

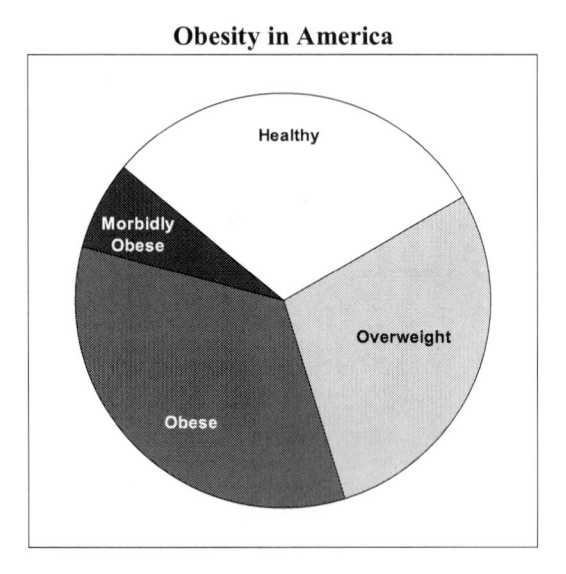

Obesity in America

According to the 2010 statistics published by the Center for Disease Control and Prevention

There really is very little public education on how to live a healthy lifestyle. It's up to us all as individuals to get educated on this topic and to share that knowledge with the people we know and care about. I hope this mini-chapter can help clear up some of the urban legends of diet.

Fact or Fiction? Carbohydrates are making Americans fat.

Fact - Americans are getting fat because highly processed carbohydrates are ubiquitous (omnipresent, being everywhere at once) in the American diet. The single leading cause of obesity, by a long shot, is too many carbs in the American diet. Eating snacks and meals with high glycemic load is literally killing us at alarming rates through diabetes and heart disease.

The stuff is everywhere. You can't avoid it randomly. You must eat very intentionally to get a properly balanced meal.

Fact or Fiction? Carbs are bad.

Fiction – A superficial understanding of carbohydrates and things like The Atkins' Revolution lead us to believe that carbs are bad. As we will discuss in the next chapter, carbohydrates are absolutely essential to your body as your main source of energy.

The problem with carbs comes when we abuse them. Our tendency is to eat too much of the wrong carbohydrates. They are cheap and easy, therefore overused. We get our carbohydrate intake under control by eating intentionally.

Fact or Fiction? Fruits are bad because they are loaded with sugar.

Fiction – Eating fruit in moderation is perfectly healthy and is a great source of micronutrients. You can go wrong by eating too much fruit, but several pieces per day is good for you. Sure, there is a lot of sugar, but there is a lot of fiber too. The fiber brings down the net carbs (net carbs = carbs – fiber) and reduces the glycemic load.

Fact or Fiction? Losing weight is simple. Eat Less, Exercise More.

Fiction – As we discussed earlier, this formula simply does not work as you might expect. Eating less lowers the metabolism, exercise more makes you hungry. These both send your brain and body the wrong message.

The right method to lose fat is to carefully eat and exercise intentionally to send your brain and body the right messages.

Fact or Fiction? Too Much Soy Protein is Bad.

Fact – Well, sort of. Soy is another one of those ubiquitous (found everywhere) foods. Processed food manufacturers love to throw fillers (like soy) in everything. Check out the labels on the food in your pantry and in your refrigerator. You will see pretty quickly that just about everything has soy. It's everywhere!

Soy comes in a few different common forms; soy lecithin, soy oil, and soy protein isolate. Read the label on any nutrition bar, protein shake, or veggie burger and you'll find soy protein listed predominantly on the list of ingredients.

Soy Protein will mess up hormones in both men and women. It increases your estrogen levels and terribly reduces your free testosterone because it is a sex hormone binding protein. These hormone imbalances will reduce your drive for healthy diet and exercise. You women have such little testosterone to begin with, you cannot afford to lose any to soy. A healthy protein blend including soy is fine.

Fact or Fiction? If you eat fat you'll get fat.

Fiction – Eating fat does not make you fat. You get fat by consuming more calories than you burn.

Fat is an essential macronutrient. You must eat fat and plenty of it. It is dense in calories, so eating fat gives you the energy you need to perform. Also, since fat is digested much slower than other nutrients, it keeps you satiated and satisfied for a longer time. Eating more fat will help you eat fewer total calories and burn more total calories.

With that said, Dr Hyman says fat comes in three categories; the good, the bad and the ugly. We'll talk more about that later.

Fact or Fiction? Too much protein is bad for you.

Fact – Just like anything else, you must eat protein in moderation. Too much protein and / or an imbalance of macronutrients can be very hard on you kidneys. Experts say 30% of your total calories is about the limit. In other words, no more than 1/3 of your diet should come from protein. In my humble opinion, no less either.

Fact or Fiction? Salt is bad.

Fiction – Sodium and other electrolytes are absolutely essential to living. Your brain will shut down, your heart will stop and you will die if you do not consume electrolytes. However, you should consume salt in moderation. Most Americans eat way too much salt.

Only about 20% of your salt intake comes from intentional use in meals and cooking. The other 80% comes from hidden sources. Restaurant food, processed food, and most of all bread are the main sources of salt in the average American diet. Cut out the processed food and the excess breads and you'll get your excess salt intake under control.

You may notice you suddenly drop 4 or 5 pounds during the first few days of dieting. That is because you tend to naturally cut back on the salt, causing you to shed water weight.

Fact or Fiction? Walking is just as good as running.

Fact – This is mostly true, depending on your goals and current condition. If you're in great shape and your goal is to increase your anaerobic threshold, then walking won't do the job. But, if you are trying to get in shape and lose weight, walking is not "just as good", it is even better than running.

Walking gets your heart going and kicks up your metabolism without sending the wrong messages or making you hungry all day. An hour per day of walking will help you race toward your weight loss goal.

Law #21 -
You must ignore all the diet misinformation.

Fact or Fiction? Diet Pills can help you lose weight and live a healthy life.

Fiction – Diet pills can literally kill you. People drop dead from some diet pills. They've caused heart valve damage and a long list of other cardiac problems. They can cause adrenal fatigue, kidney problems, and serious hormonal imbalances. Worst of all, diet pills are counterproductive because they lead to a significantly reduced metabolism and yoyo dieting.

Please stay away from diet pills. Sure they may come from a doctor, but that doesn't make them safe.

Fact or Fiction? I just need to go on a diet to lose some weight.

Fiction – Ask any overweight person and they will agree; going on a diet may help with short term weight loss, but does nothing for long term weight loss and health. It takes much more than just going on a diet. You must live a healthy lifestyle with an appropriate healthy diet for life, with plenty of exercise.

It's not just one thing, it is everything. You have to change the way you think and the way you live.

Fact or Fiction? Processed food is bad.

Fact – Yes, yes, yes, processed food is horrible for you. We will discuss whole food in detail later, but for now you need to know that processed food is bad for you. The closer you are to the original source the better. Food should come from farms, not factories.

Fact or Fiction? Fat people just have a slow metabolism.

Fiction – Well, mostly fiction anyway. You are in complete control of your own metabolism. With appropriate diet and exercise your metabolism will rev up like a super star.

Fact or Fiction? You shouldn't weigh yourself every day.

Fiction – I'm a data guy; I love data. I already told you to track everything. How are you going to do that if you are not taking measurements? Weigh yourself, collect the data; track it and log it.

Now here is where most people get into trouble… You can't worry about the actual daily numbers and what they mean. You only care about the overall trend. You'll have days that are flat and days that you go up and days that you go down. None of that matters as long as your trend is always going in the right direction.

Let the trend be your friend.

Take a look below at this screen shot from MyFitnessPal. There are ups and downs. Good days and bad. But the overall trend is down.

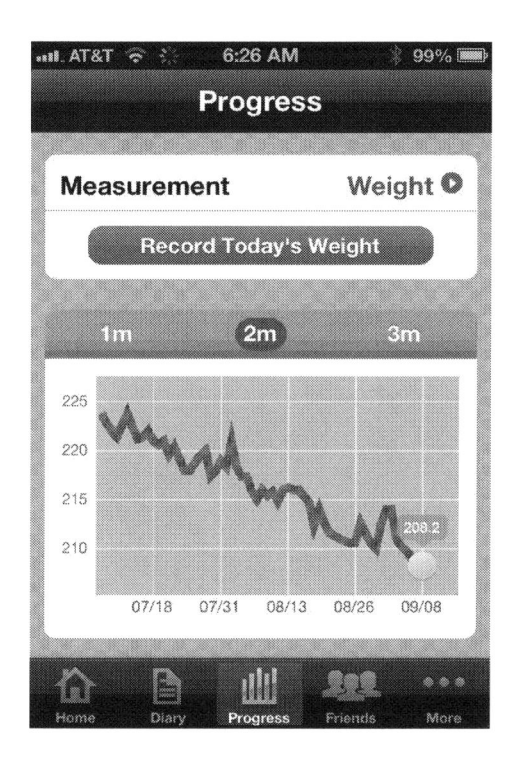

Fact or Fiction? Group setting diet programs will help you lose weight.

Fiction – Group setting diet programs have a horrible long term success rate. Sure, you might be the one out of 500 who is successful, but the odds are against you.

The problem is not the group setting; to the contrary, having accountability is helpful. The problem is these programs are dieting-centric. You can't have permanent weight loss by going on a diet. It takes a permanent lifestyle change. Be accountable to yourself. Be accountable to your daily lifestyle choices for life, not just Tuesday before the meeting, not just for the next three months.

Fact or Fiction? Artificial sweetens are bad for you.

Fact – Yes, they are very bad! Just Google "artificial sweeteners" and you can learn all about it. Basically, everybody in the world except for the food lobby and the US Government agrees. The rich and powerful food companies manipulate the government and the people in order to keep shoving these poisons down our throats. Why? Because it is profitable. Not because they are evil, but because you want to buy it!

They'll probably sue me for this paragraph and take all the proceeds from this book. I don't care, you deserve the truth.

There is a fairly new product on the market that is a zero calorie natural sweetener made from the **Stevia Leaf**. This is not an artificial sweetener. We are still in the early days, but it seems that stevia may be a healthy alternative to sugar and artificial sweeteners. The jury is still out, but I'm leaning toward giving stevia my seal of approval.

Fact or Fiction? Diet food and "heath food" will help you lose weight.

Fiction – Most diet food and even "health food" is just processed factory food, filled with soy protein, salt and other fillers. You can't have permanent weight loss unless you switch to a healthy diet for life. Balance your nutrients and ditch the processed food. Processed food with some healthy sounding name is still processed food.

One personal exception for me is the brand name "Amy's Kitchen". It is not exactly whole food, but it is as close as you can get in the frozen food section.

Fact or Fiction? A calorie is a calorie.

Fiction – Nothing could be further from the truth. The quality of the food is much more important than the number of calories. On one hand, I like to use calories as a simple method for monitoring food quantities. On the other hand, I know that calories are a bogus red herring that can easily distract you from what is really important, food quality.

Eating 1300 calories of processed foods per day will make you fat. However, eating 2500 calories of wholesome food per day will keep you lean. For example, a scoop of ice cream has nearly the same amount of fat and calories as a scoop of guacamole. The guacamole will make you lean, while the ice cream will not.

Fact or Fiction? Eating out is OK as long as you are careful.

Fiction – This one is pretty tricky. As long as you eat the right food at the right times, in the right quantities, it doesn't matter too much if it comes from the farm, the grocery or a restaurant. The problem is that most restaurants sneak in some not so good choices that you are unaware of.

They add lots of extra salt. They use the wrong selection of oils based on cost and taste rather than health and nutrition. The portion sizes are too big, they always have more calories than you think and they tend to over use the carbohydrates. They usually don't cook using the healthiest practices that you would choose at home.

So, I guess you could in fact eat healthy at restaurants. But I warn you, it is difficult. Use MyFitnessPal to check out your meal before you order.

Forget what you've heard.

As you can see, there are lots of misconceptions and false understandings about eating healthy. Don't fall into these common traps. Ignore the scuttlebutt and the rumors by getting your information from a reliable source.

Chapter 13 - Macronutrients

Pay close attention because this chapter is probably the most important chapter in the book. Everything else was leading up to this critical point. Everything in this book so far teaches you general principles about living a healthy lifestyle, but in this chapter we get into the details of what a healthy diet actually is.

MICRO-nutrients are needed by your body to live. These are the small trace elements and substances found in food. We are talking about vitamins and minerals, and all the little chemicals that make us tick. Micronutrients are found in everything we eat to varying degrees and are a critical part of our diet. However, these micronutrients are a very small part of our diets. The vast bulk of what we eat are macronutrients.

MACRO-nutrients make up the majority of everything you consume. They are our source of energy and the building blocks from which our body is made. When they say "You are what you eat", it is literally true. The macronutrients you eat are absorbed by and become part of your body. You really are what you eat.

The three macronutrients your body requires are:
- Carbohydrates
- Fats
- Proteins

All three are absolutely essential and required for life.

Balanced Diet
The term "balanced diet" has been so overused and cliché that we have lost track of the actual meaning. The absolute number one most important rule in this book is...

Law #22 -
You must have a balanced diet. Balance your macronutrients.

It is critically important that you have the appropriate amounts of all three macronutrients, every meal, every day. Having a balanced diet means that you've balanced your macronutrients.

The old way recommends a "healthy diet" with 65% of your calories coming from carbohydrates, with only 15% coming from protein and 20% coming from fat. Most contemporary nutritionists agree this old method is great (for getting fat). This diet is way too high in carbohydrates.

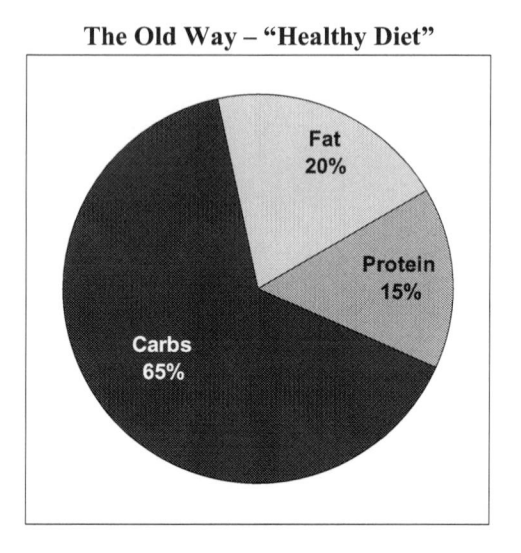

The Old Way – "Healthy Diet"

- Carbs 65%
- Fat 20%
- Protein 15%

Now we recommend 40% carbohydrates, 30% protein and 30% fats. That means no more than 40% of your daily calorie intake should come from carbs. The new method is to decrease your carbs and increase your protein and fat.

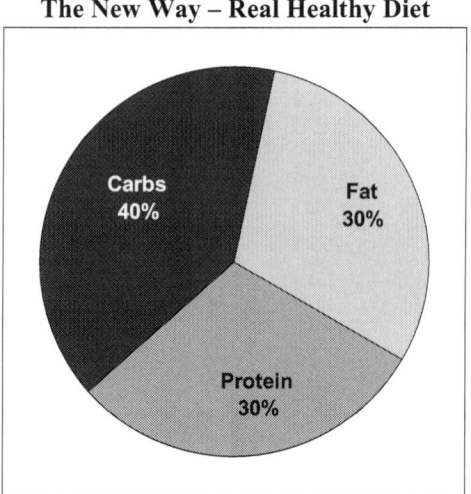

The New Way – Real Healthy Diet

- Carbs 40%
- Fat 30%
- Protein 30%

Diet – Macronutrients 69

You can use an application like MyFitnessPal to monitor these numbers on a daily basis. Here is a screen shot from the smart phone app.

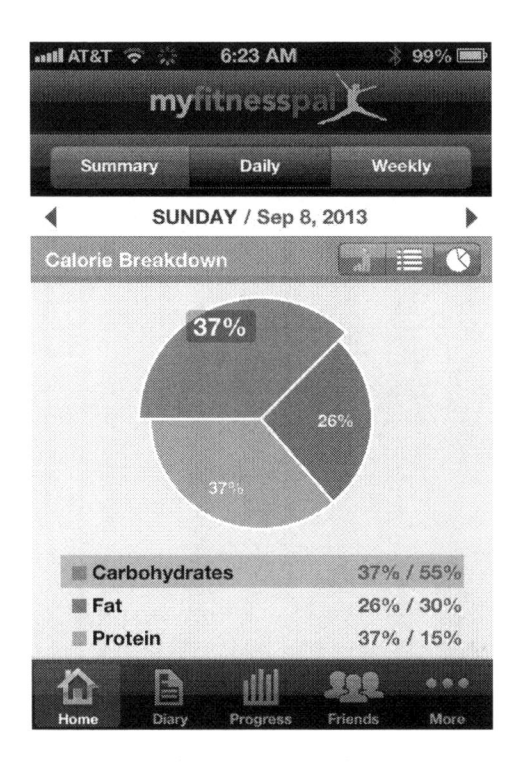

Law #23 -
Your calories should be 40% Carb, 30% Protein & 30% Fat.

Maintain this healthy ratio during every meal for optimal health and nutrition.

Protein

Proteins are molecules made up from amino acids. This is the most neglected of all macronutrients. Protein has a bad reputation because it is associated with greasy red meats which are heavy in saturated fats. However, protein comes from all kinds of healthy foods.

You are made of protein. Your tissue, muscles, organs and part of every cell in your body are protein. The protein from the foods we eat gets digested and broken down into amino acids. Those amino acids are then used to build you. You are what you eat, and in this case, it is quite literal. Your body is the reassembled amino acids from the food you eat.

Proteins come from a wide variety of sources like:
- Meats, beef, ham, pork, poultry and fish
- Legumes like beans & peas: black beans, chickpeas, pinto beans
- Eggs, cheese and dairy
- Nuts and Seeds: almonds, cashews, peanuts, walnuts, pumpkin seeds
- Fruits and Vegetables: spinach, soy, mushrooms, broccoli, asparagus, etc.
- Supplements like Whey Protein Powder, Casein Protein Powder, etc.

Were you surprised to see fruits and vegetables on the list? Don't be. Some vegetables are loaded with protein. Just about every food you can eat has a mix of all three macronutrients. Take almonds for example. 100 grams of almonds has 19.5 grams of protein, 6.2 grams of carbohydrates and 52 grams of fat.

So are almonds a protein, a carb or a fat? They are all three, just like most every other food.

You will see that some foods are heavy in protein, heavy in carbohydrates or heavy in fat. You will see that some foods are pretty well balanced all by themselves. It is up to you to select the right food choices to balance every meal.

For example, a turkey breast sandwich with mayo is perfect because it has all three macronutrients in the correct proportions.

One consideration is that most plant proteins (other than soy beans) are incomplete proteins, while animal based proteins are considered complete proteins. As such, you may need to eat complimenting foods in order to create the complete proteins you need for good nutrition. For example, rice and beans are each incomplete, but together form a complete protein.

The point of all this protein talk is not to get you to load up on protein. It is to get you to understand what proportion of protein is right for a healthy diet. Too much protein will damage your kidneys and hinder your metabolism, too little will make you fat (or maybe skinny-fat).

Take a look at the table on the next page. The data was collected from FoodNutritionTable.com, a great online source for nutritional information. In the table you will see nutritional information from some common foods. Observe the proportions of each macronutrient.

Another word of caution about soy protein. I avoid it. For me, soy protein was the difference between losing fat and plateauing. Soy is a "sex hormone binding protein" and will eat up your free testosterone and make you over produce estrogen. This is great for building a feminine curvy body, but not so great for being lean.

That reduction in testosterone will suck up all your energy, leaving you as a couch potato. And if you read the label, couch potatoes are filled with fat. If you want to be leaner, cut out the soy protein. At least cut back; if soy protein is listed as one of the top three ingredients, take a pass.

Diet – Macronutrients

Food Per 100 grams	Calories	Protein grams	Carbs grams	Fat grams	Fiber grams	Net Carbs
Almonds	583	19.5	6.2	52	10.6	0
Apple	54	0.4	12	0	2.3	9.7
Asparagus	17	1.9	1.3	0.2	1.5	0
Avocados	188	2.6	1.5	18.1	6.4	0
Bacon	882	0.2	0	99.7	0	0
Bagel - Sour Dough	313	10	55	5.1	2.5	52.5
Bass	87	15	0	3	0	0
Beef Rib eye	146	22.8	0.2	6	0	0.2
Beef Tenderloin	116	23.7	0	2.3	0	0
Black Beans	154	9	24	0.5	8.5	15.5
Bread - White	255	9.2	45	3.5	2.5	42.5
Bread - Wheat	266	8.2	48.8	3	4.7	44.1
Broccoli	29	3.3	2	0.2	3.5	0
Butter	735	0.7	0.7	82.5	0	0.7
Carrots	27	0.8	4.7	0	2.9	1.8
Cashews	591	18.5	22.5	46.5	7.5	15
Cauliflower	24	2	3	0	2.2	0.8
Celery	17	0.7	3.5	0.1	1.6	1.9
Cheddar Cheese	389	25.4	0.5	32.2	0	0.5
Chicken Breast	100	22.8	0	0.9	0	0
Chicken Dark Meat	103	20.6	0	2.3	0	0
Chickpeas	119	7.5	13	3	5.4	7.6
Cola	44	0	11	0	0	11
Corn	354	9.2	65.5	3.8	9.2	56.3
Cottage Cheese	100	12.8	2.9	4.2	0	2.9
Crab	85	17	1	1.4	0	1
Doughnut	440	4.5	50	24.5	1.5	48.5
Egg	139	12.5	0	10	0	0
Egg White	49	11.1	0.7	0.2	0	0.7
Endive	19	1.5	1	0	3.5	0
Flour Tortilla	94	2.49	15.4	2.32	0.9	14.5

Diet – Macronutrients

Food Per 100 grams	Calories	Protein grams	Carbs grams	Fat grams	Fiber grams	Net Carbs
Grapes	57	0.5	13.5	0	0.5	13
Green Beans	36	2.4	6	0.3	3.5	2.5
Ham	136	17.4	1.5	6.8	0	1.5
Hamburger	272	21	2.5	20	0	2.5
Hoggie Roll	282	8.5	50	4.5	2.8	47.2
Lemon	36	0.5	6.5	0.4	2.2	4.3
Macadamia Nuts	733	9	6.5	74.5	6.5	0
Milk - reduced fat	46	3.4	4.8	1.5	0	4.8
Milk - Whole	62	3.7	4.3	3.4	0	4.3
Mushrooms	16	2.7	0.3	0	2.5	0
Orange	44	1	9.5	0.2	2.1	7.4
Pancakes	210	7.6	30	6.5	0.5	29.5
Pasta	359	13.5	67	3	3.4	63.6
Peanut Butter	625	26	12	52	6	6
Pork tenderloin	119	22.8	0	3.1	0	0
Potato Chips	557	5.5	43	39.5	6	37
Potatoes	85	2	17.6	0.1	2.6	15
Pumpkin	36	1.1	7	0.2	1	6
Pumpkin Seeds	345	24.6	7	23.5	5.4	1.6
Rice - Brown	137	3.2	26	1.5	3	23
Rice - White	96	2.5	20	0.4	0.8	19.2
Soybeans	428	37	29.5	18	5	24.5
Spinach	15	2.5	0.6	0.3	2	0
Strawberries	36	0.8	6.5	0.4	2	4.5
Sweet Potato	96	1.3	21	0.1	2.5	18.5
Tortilla Chips	509	7.1	66.5	23.6	1.1	65.4
Trout	126	18.4	0	5.8	0	0
Tuna	96	21.5	0	1	0	0
Turkey Breast	106	22.6	0.6	1.4	0	0.6
Walnuts	675	14.4	12.1	62.5	8	4.1
Yogurt	65	3.8	4.5	3.5	0	4.5

Carbohydrates

Carbohydrates are a large group of organic compounds found in food that include sugars, starch and cellulose. Just like the other two macronutrients, carbohydrates are essential to healthy living.

Food labels itemize carbs into three categories of total carbohydrates, sugar and fiber. That's important because of the way carbs are metabolized by the body. Looking at these numbers we can infer the Glycemic Index of the food.

The "sugars" essentially go straight into the blood. But fiber slows the rate at which the sugars are metabolized.

Net Carbs

I have mentioned net carbs several times now. Net carbs are calculated as total carbohydrates minus dietary fiber. Since the fiber is not really metabolized and used for energy, it simply does not get counted. Dietary fiber is a carbohydrate, but is nutritionally different than other carbohydrates.

In the same way fiber is a special kind of carbohydrate, so is sugar. Fiber is not counted, but sugar should almost be counted twice! The sugar in the food you eat rushes to your blood stream and causes an insulin response. We use the Glycemic Index to measure the affect.

Glycemic Index and Glycemic Load

The glycemic index (GI) tells you how fast blood glucose rises after eating a specific food. Some sugary foods have very high glycemic index, while non-carbohydrate food has a very low glycemic index. In other words, the glycemic index tells you how sugary a food is and if you will be riding the insulin roller coaster.

Glycemic Index Guidelines

Low GI	55 or less	Beans, legumes, seeds, nuts, most fruits and vegetables.
Medium GI	56 to 69	Whole grains, potatoes, some fruits.
High GI	70 and above.	White bread, white rice, corn products, most cakes and candy.

Glycemic load takes into account the quantity of the food, where glycemic index does not. Or more importantly, the glycemic load of a food or a meal takes into account all of the elements of the meal. You can have small amounts of high glycemic index foods without having a particularly high glycemic load meal.

Law #24 -
A healthy diet has a low glycemic load.

The White Menace
The White Menace is sugar. When we talk about food with a high glycemic index, it is all white (or brown once you deep fry it).

So as a rule, stay away from food that is white or can be white. Sugar, flour, bread, potatoes, ice cream and rice are all high glycemic index foods. These foods should make up the minority of your diet, or avoided all together.

Eating too many white carbs will cause you to get fat and have serious medical issues like heart disease. You'll be riding the insulin rollercoaster again, leading to Metabolic Syndrome and eventually Diabetes.

High Fructose Corn Syrup
High Fructose Corn Syrup (HFCS) is an industrially processed food. When you see it on a label you should consider it a big red flag that you are about to eat a highly processed, high glycemic index, low quality, factory food. It is a sugar product that is not found in nature because it is only made in food laboratories. In my "opinion", it is literally one of the worst carbohydrates you can eat, because it is both high glycemic index and highly processed.

The corn industry will tell you there is nothing wrong with HFCS. But don't believe them. HFCS is bad news!

Fats

The BIG myth related to fat is the idea that eating fat makes you fat; this is simply not true. This idea that we should be eating a low fat diet is just wrong minded. Fat is a critical macronutrient needed for healthy living, and should not be avoided. For that matter, fats should make up a full 30% of your healthy diet.

There are several important benefits to eating fat (other than the fact that you will die of malnutrition if you don't)

- Fat makes you feel full. Sometimes it is hard to feel satiated, especially with a high carb, low fat diet. You just feel hungry all the time. Kick up the fat intake and that feeling will go away.

- Fat digests slowly, making you feel fuller longer. Ever eat a salad or some lean chicken only to be hungry again in an hour. Fat will slow that process down and have you feeling fuller longer.

- Eating fat gives you long lasting energy. The calorie density of fat is very high. You might think that is bad because you want to stay away from high calorie food. However, with this densely packed nutrient, a little goes a long way.

Now that I've finished telling you how great fat is, let me give you the bad news. Some fats are good and healthy for you, some fats are not so good for you, and other fats are downright toxic. Let's take a look at the different types of fat.

Keep in mind that most foods have multiple different fats, but tend to be higher in one or another. For instance, 100 grams of Sesame Oil has 16 grams of saturated fat, 42 grams of monounsaturated and 42 grams of polyunsaturated.

Omega 3 Fatty Acid - Great

Omega-3 is the best fat for your nutrition (in moderation, like everything else). It is an essential fatty acid found in"

- Fish oils: Anchovies, algae, squid, krill.
- Plants, Nuts and Seeds: Flax seed oil, Hemp oil, kiwi, chia seed, black raspberry, canola, hazel nuts, pecan,

Not exactly a vast selection. That's why you might consider an Omega-3 Supplement like fish oil or flaxseed oil. Even then, it is difficult to find a high quality supplement. Read your labels.

Monounsaturated Fat - Good
Monounsaturated fats are good for you, they help you stay happy and healthy

- Avocados
- Olives
- Pumpkin Seeds
- Sesame Seeds
- Olive Oil
- Sunflower Oil
- Sesame Oil
- Almond Oil
- Hazelnuts
- Almonds
- Cashews
- Peanut Butter

Going back to FoodNutritionTable.com you can see the breakdown of all the different types of fats in your favorite foods.

Polyunsaturated - Omega 6 Fatty Acid - Good
Polyunsaturated along with monounsaturated fat, make up the healthy unsaturated fats. Polyunsaturated fat is good for you, and easily found in lots of foods.

- Seafood
- Wheat Germs
- Cucumber
- Safflower Oil
- Corn Oil
- Soy Oil
- Nuts and Seeds
- Walnuts
- Linseed Oil

Saturated Fat - Bad
Saturated fats are not particularly good for you. They tend to clog your arteries and harm your cardiac health. Saturated fat comes from some nuts and most meat and poultry. The variety of saturated fat found in nuts and seeds is not as bad for you as the saturated fats found in meat, but unsaturated fat is certainly preferred.

- Beef
- Pork
- Lamb
- Chicken Legs
- Turkey Legs
- Duck
- Coconut Oil
- Mayonnaise
- Palm Oil

Just like anything else, saturated fat is not too bad for you in moderation. The problems occur when you eat excess saturated fat. You can eat it; just keep it to a minimum. You might want to skip the T-Bone and select a lean cut of filet instead. Limit the red meat to one portion per week and perhaps lean poultry only once per day. *Just a little side note: saturated fats are a main contributor to acid reflux.*

We will talk more about this topic in the section on Vegetarianism later in the book.

Trans Fat - Toxic
Trans fat is the Frankenstein of fats. Not found in nature, this fat is fabricated in food laboratories. Fats naturally spoil, just like all organic food products. Scientists thought, "Wouldn't it be great if we could make food that never went bad?" Thus the genesis of trans fat. By hydrogenating oil they were able to dramatically increase the shelf life of any food product.

Here's the problem... Food spoils as it is being eaten by microorganisms. The only way to get food not to spoil is by making it so toxic microorganisms won't eat it. Those same microorganisms are in your gut (biotics) as a big part of digestion.

Take a scoop of Margarine (trans fat) and a scoop of butter and put them both outside on the sidewalk. Watch as the ants eat the butter, but walk around the margarine. Why? Because it is toxic!

We humans are supposed to be the smart ones. The microorganisms and the ants have figured this out, but we can't seem to understand; don't eat food that was made in a laboratory. Read the label, if it says:

- Trans Fat
- Hydrogenated
- Partially Hydrogenated

Don't eat it. It doesn't matter that the jar of peanut butter has a big label on the front that says "No Trans Fat". When you read the nutritional label it says "partially hydrogenated peanut oil". Read your labels. Don't eat it.

Trans Fat is another food product that makes me wag my finger at the government. This ought to be a banned substance instead of fully integrated into our food supply. Lobbyist and campaign contributions at work!

But again, this entire section on trans-fat is just my "opinion".

By the way, if a product has less than a half gram of fat per serving, they can legally call it zero! So if your spray butter serving size is ½ gram and it is literally 100% fat, they can say on the label "Contains Zero Fat!"

Chapter 14 - Dietary Worksheet

There are lots of equations and information in this book. The following worksheet will help you put it all together. You can do most of this worksheet now, but you might need to come back to it after reading the chapters on fitness and exercise.

This worksheet might look a little daunting at first, but don't worry I'll walk you through it. It is all easy math, and you can always look at the examples for extra help. There are example forms already filled out after this blank form. So if you get a little confused just look at one of the examples.

Grab your pencil (not a pen) and a calculator and let's get started on the next page.

We'll start off by calculating your Lean Body Mass (LBM). As we discussed, this is your weight minus the weight of your fat. The formulas are an approximation and can be off by a little.

Weight: You need to grab a scale and measure your weight in pounds. Optimally, weigh yourself naked, first thing in the morning, before you eat or drink anything.

Ladies - Wrist: Use the tape measure to measure around your wrist at the most narrow point on your arm. Take the measurement in inches.

Ladies - Forearm: Using the tape measure, measure around your forearm at the thickest point between your elbow and your hand. Take the measurement in inches.

Waist: Measure around your waist at the belly button. It doesn't matter where you wear your pants, this measurement happens around your midsection, right across your belly button. Take the measurement in inches.

Ladies - Hip: Measure around your booty at the widest point, right around your butt and pelvis. Take the measurement in inches.

Equation for LBM: Take each of your measurements and multiply them by the factor listed to the right. Add and subtract the products to calculate your Lean Body Mass. Pay attention to the signs; some numbers get added in while others are subtracted out.

Next we calculate Body Fat Percentage. We subtract your LBM from your total weight, multiply by one hundred, divide by your weight and voilà, you have %BF.

Dietary Worksheet – Page 1

Men

Body weight:
W._____ pounds

Waist circumference:
B._____ inches

Lean Body Mass:
+   W._____ x 1.082 = _____
−   B._____ x 4.15 = _____
                     +   94.42
=   LBM: _____

Percentage Body Fat:
    W._____ − LBM._____
x   100 _____
÷   W. _____
=   %BF _____

Women

Body weight in pounds:
W._____ pounds

Wrist circumference:
C._____ inches

Forearm circumference:
F._____ inches

Waist circumference:
B._____ inches

Hip circumference:
E._____ inches

Lean Body Mass:
+   W._____ x 0.732 = _____
+   C._____ x 0.318 = _____
+   F._____ x 0.434 = _____
−   B._____ x 0.157 = _____
−   E._____ x 0.249 = _____
                     +   8.987
=   LBM: _____

Percentage Body Fat:
    W._____ − LBM._____
x   100 _____
÷   W. _____
=   %BF _____

Diet – Dietary Worksheet

Basal Metabolic Rate is the total number of calories you burn just being alive. Whether you're sitting on the couch, at your desk or lying in bed, you are constantly burning calories. That number of calories is called your BMR.

Multiply your Lean Body Mass by 13.8 and that number is your BMR in calories.

In addition to your BMR, you burn more calories during activity. Let's add up the number of hours you spend working out. We break it up into hours per week of light, medium and vigorous exercise.

Light Exercise: This is stuff like fast walking, water aerobics, swimming, etc. This does not include you being on your feet at work or walking around your office. It only counts if you get your heart rate elevated above 60% of your max heart rate.

Medium Exercise: Hours per week of cycling, fast swimming, light jogging, etc. These are activities that get your heart rate up above 70% of your max.

Vigorous Exercise: Hours per week of intense training, interval training, running, Insanity Workout, etc. These are the exercises that get your heart rate up above 82% of maximum.

Add up the hours to get the total number of exercise hours per week.

Notice I did not include weight training. You do burn calories while weight training, however the number is already included in your BMR because it effects your LBM.

Calculate your approximate Maximum Heart Rate (MaxHR) by subtracting your age from 220. This formula is more or less correct, but you need a stress test to find the actual number. I'm 40 years old and my max HR is 191 beats per minute, significantly higher than the 180 BPM estimated by the equation.

Calculate your average heart rate during exercise based on your max heart rate and time training in each heart rate zone. (We talk more about heart rate training in the chapters on exercise)

Dietary Worksheet – Page 2

Basal Metabolic Rate:

LBM _____ x 13.8 = BMR _____

Activity:

Hours of light exercise per week (fast walking)   H1 _____

Hours of medium exercise per week (cycling)   H2 _____

Hours of vigorous exercise per week (Intervals)   H4 _____

H1 _____ + H2 _____ + H4 _____ = H_{Sum} _____

Heart Rate:

220 – Age _____ = HR_{Max} _____ BPM

HR_{Max} _____ x 0.60 = HR1 _____ BPM

HR_{Max} _____ x 0.71 = HR2 _____ BPM

HR_{Max} _____ x 0.82 = HR4 _____ BPM

HR_{Avg}:

  HR1 _____ x H1 _____ = _____ BPM

+ HR2 _____ x H2 _____ = _____ BPM

+ HR4 _____ x H4 _____ = _____ BPM

= _____ ÷ H_{Sum} = HR_{Avg} _____

Let's now calculate the calories burned during exercise. Put your weight, average heart rate from the previous page and your age to calculate "Temp". Multiply "Temp" by the total number of hours of exercise per week from the previous page, multiplied by 2.05 to get the average number of calories burned per day during exercise.

Total Daily Calories Burned is the number of calories for all activities. Take your BMR and Calories burned during activity to find your total calories burned.
*BMR is calculated using the Sterling-Pasmore Equation

Now let's consider losing weight. If you intend on losing weight, you'll need a short term diet which has a calorie deficiency. You'll need to come back and redo this worksheet again once you've reached your healthy weight and periodically during your weight loss process. (For me, that was over several years)

Enter in your desired weight loss per week in pounds. If you want to lose 1 pound of fat per week, enter WL = 1. If you want to exchange 1 pound of fat for 1 pound of muscle, enter WL = 0 because your total weight change per week needs to be zero. You might go with WL = 1.0 or even 1.5 pounds of fat loss per week, but please don't go any higher.

"D" stands for Deficiency. Your Deficiency is the total number of calories per day you need to be deficient in order to lose the desired fat, considering your weight loss goals, 7 days per week at 3500 calories per pound.

Subtract your required deficiency from your total daily calorie burn to find the number of calories you should eat daily for your desired weight loss goals.

Dietary Worksheet – Page 3

Calories Burned During Activity:

Men	Women
Age _____ x 0.2 = _____	Age _____ x 0.074 = _____
+ HR_{Avg} _____ x 0.63 = _____	+ HR_{Avg} _____ x 0.45 = _____
+ W. _____ x 0.09 = _____	− W. _____ x 0.057 = _____
− 55	− 20.4
= Temp _____	= Temp _____

Temp _____ x H_{Sum} _____ x 2.05 = Cal_{Act} _____

Total Daily Calories Burned:

BMR _____ + Cal_{Act} _____ = Cal_B _____

Desired Weight Change per Week: WL = _____

Daily Calorie Deficiency: WL _____ x 3500 ÷ 7 = D _____

Daily Calorie Consumption – For Fat Loss:

Cal_B _____ − D _____ = Cal_D _____

We calculated your total daily calorie needs on the previous page. Let's use that information to find your required macronutrient intake.

Considering 40% of your total calories coming from Carbs, 30% Protein and 30% Fat, calculate the number of calories for each macronutrient.

Considering a gram of carbohydrates and a gram of protein each contain about 4 calories, and a gram of fat contains about 9 calories, calculate the number of grams you require of each macronutrient.

That's it... Now you know what to eat.

This was not just an exercise; this is you calculating your nutritional needs. These are your numbers, stick to them for maximum success for your personal weight goal. Don't forget to recalculate from time to time as your goals and weight loss needs change.

Dietary Worksheet – Page 4

Macronutrient Calories per Day:

Calories from Carbs: = Cal_D _____ x 0.4 = Cal_C _____ calories

Calories from Protein: = Cal_D _____ x 0.3 = Cal_P _____ calories

Calories from Fat: = Cal_D _____ x 0.3 = Cal_F _____ calories

Grams of Macronutrients per Day:

Grams of Carbohydrates   = Cal_C _____ ÷ 4 = _____ grams

Grams of Protein   = Cal_P _____ ÷ 4 = _____ grams

Grams of Fat   = Cal_F _____ ÷ 9 = _____ grams

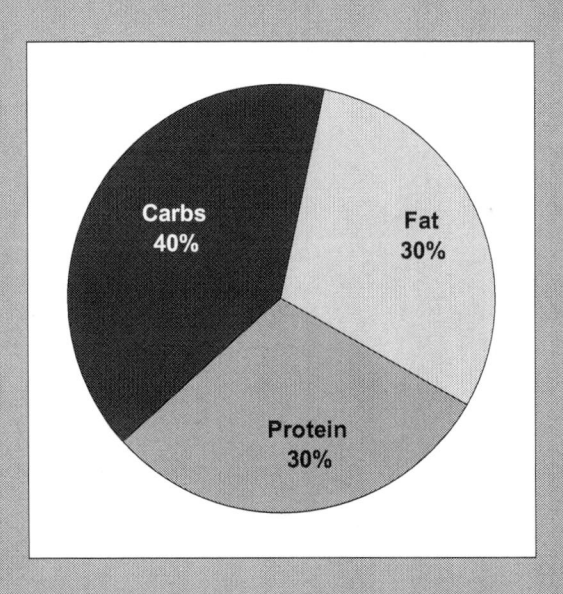

Diet – Dietary Worksheet

So let's take a look at the form when it is filled out and completed. We'll do an example as a man, followed by an example as a woman.

Male Example - Dietary Worksheet – Page 1

Men	Women
Body weight:	Body weight in pounds:
W. __207__ pounds	W. _____ pounds
Waist circumference:	Wrist circumference:
B. __38.25__ inches	C. _____ inches
	Forearm circumference:
	F. _____ inches
	Waist circumference:
	B. _____ inches
	Hip circumference:
	E. _____ inches
Lean Body Mass:	Lean Body Mass:
+ W. __207__ x 1.082 = __224__	+ W. _____ x 0.732 = _____
− B. __38.25__ x 4.15 = __158.7__	+ C. _____ x 0.318 = _____
+ 94.42	+ F. _____ x 0.434 = _____
= LBM: __159.7__	− B. _____ x 0.157 = _____
	− E. _____ x 0.249 = _____
	+ 8.987
	= LBM: _____
Percentage Body Fat:	Percentage Body Fat:
W. __207__ − LBM. __159.7__	W. _____ − LBM. _____
x 100 __4730__	x 100 _____
÷ W. __207__	÷ W. _____
= %BF __22.85 %__	= %BF _____

Male Example - Dietary Worksheet – Page 2

Basal Metabolic Rate:

LBM __**159.7**__ x 13.8 = BMR __**2204 calories**__

Activity:

Hours of light exercise per week (fast walking)   H1 __**4**__
Hours of medium exercise per week (cycling)   H2 __**1.5**__
Hours of vigorous exercise per week (Intervals)   H4 __**0.75**__

H1 __**4**__ + H2 __**1.5**__ + H4 __**0.75**__ = H_{Sum} __**6.25**__

Heart Rate:

220 – Age __**40**__ = HR_{Max} __**180**__ BPM

HR_{Max} __**180**__ x 0.60 = HR1 __**108**__ BPM
HR_{Max} __**180**__ x 0.71 = HR2 __**128**__ BPM
HR_{Max} __**180**__ x 0.82 = HR4 __**148**__ BPM

HR_{Avg}:

   HR1 __**108**__ x H1 __**4**__ = __**432**__ BPM
+ HR2 __**128**__ x H2 __**1.5**__ = __**192**__ BPM
+ HR4 __**148**__ x H4 __**0.75**__ = __**111**__ BPM

= __**735**__ ÷ H_{Sum} = HR_{Avg} __**118**__

Male Example - Dietary Worksheet – Page 3

Calories Burned During Activity:

	Men				Women		
	Age __40__ x 0.2	= __8__			Age ____ x 0.074	= ____	
+	HR_{Avg} __118__ x 0.63	= __74__		+	HR_{Avg} ____ x 0.45	= ____	
+	W. __207__ x 0.09	= __18.6__		−	W. ____ x 0.057	= ____	
		− 55				− 20.4	
=		Temp __45.6__		=		Temp ____	

Temp __45.6__ x H_{Sum} __6.25__ x 2.05 = Cal_{Act} __584__

Total Daily Calories Burned:

BMR __2204__ + Cal_{Act} __584__ = Cal_B __2788__

Desired Weight Change per Week: WL = __1__

Daily Calorie Deficiency: WL __1__ x 3500 ÷ 7 = D __500__

Daily Calorie Consumption – For Fat Loss:

Cal_B __2788__ − D __500__ = Cal_D __2288 Calories / Day__

Male Example - Dietary Worksheet – Page 4

Macronutrient Calories per Day:

Calories from Carbs: = Cal_D __**2288**__ x 0.4 = Cal_C __**915**__ calories

Calories from Protein: = Cal_D __**2288**__ x 0.3 = Cal_P __**686**__ calories

Calories from Fat: = Cal_D __**2288**__ x 0.3 = Cal_F __**686**__ calories

Grams of Macronutrients per Day:

Grams of Carbohydrates = Cal_C __**915**__ ÷ 4 = __**229**__ grams

Grams of Protein = Cal_P __**686**__ ÷ 4 = __**171**__ grams

Grams of Fat = Cal_F __**686**__ ÷ 9 = __**76**__ grams

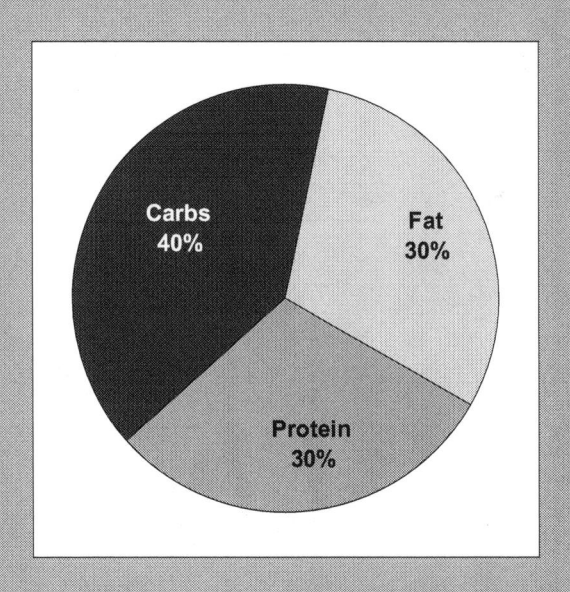

94   Diet – Dietary Worksheet

Now we'll go through the worksheet one more time as a woman. *No need to put on a dress fellas.*

Female Example - Dietary Worksheet – Page 1

Men	**Women**
Body weight: W. _____ pounds	Body weight in pounds: W. **215** pounds
Waist circumference at belly button: B. _____ inches	Wrist circumference: C. **7.5** inches Forearm circumference: F. **10.5** inches Waist circumference at belly button: B. **49** inches Hip circumference: E. **48** inches

Lean Body Mass:
+ W. _____ x 1.082 = _____
− B. _____ x 4.15 = _____
                + 94.42
= LBM: _____
	Lean Body Mass:
	+ W. **215** x 0.732 = **157**
	+ C. **7.5** x 0.318 = **2.4**
	+ F. **10.5** x 0.434 = **4.6**
	− B. **49** x 0.157 = **7.7**
	− E. **48** x 0.249 = **12**
	                + 8.987
	= LBM: **153.3**

Percentage Body Fat:
    W. _____ − LBM. _____
x 100 _____
÷ W. _____
= %BF _____
	Percentage Body Fat:
	    W. **215** − LBM. **153.3**
	x 100 **6170**
	÷ W. **215**
	= %BF **28.7 %**

Female Example - Dietary Worksheet – Page 2

Basal Metabolic Rate:

LBM **153.3** x 13.8 = BMR **2115 calories**

Activity:

Hours of light exercise per week (fast walking)	H1	**4**
Hours of medium exercise per week (cycling)	H2	**1.5**
Hours of vigorous exercise per week (Intervals)	H4	**0.75**

H1 **4** + H2 **1.5** + H4 **0.75** = H_{Sum} **6.25**

Heart Rate:

220 – Age **40** = HR_{Max} **180** BPM

HR_{Max} **180** x 0.60 = HR1 **108** BPM

HR_{Max} **180** x 0.71 = HR2 **128** BPM

HR_{Max} **180** x 0.82 = HR4 **148** BPM

HR_{Avg}:

   HR1 **108** x H1 **4** = **432** BPM

+ HR2 **128** x H2 **1.5** = **192** BPM

+ HR4 **148** x H4 **0.75** = **111** BPM

= **735** ÷ H_{Sum} = HR_{Avg} **118**

Female Example - Dietary Worksheet – Page 3

Calories Burned During Activity:

Men	Women
Age _____ x 0.2 = _____	Age **40** x 0.074 = **3**
+ HR_{Avg} _____ x 0.63 = _____	+ HR_{Avg} **118** x 0.45 = **53**
+ W. _____ x 0.09 = _____	− W. **215** x 0.057 = **12**
− 55	− 20.4
= Temp _____	= Temp **23.6**

Temp **23.6** x H_{Sum} **6.25** x 2.05 = Cal_{Act} **302**

Total Daily Calories Burned:

BMR **2115** + Cal_{Act} **302** = Cal_B **2417**

Desired Weight Change per Week: WL = **1**
Daily Calorie Deficiency: WL **1** x 3500 ÷ 7 = D **500**

Daily Calorie Consumption – For Fat Loss:

Cal_B **2417** − D **500** = Cal_D **1917 Calories / Day**

Female Example - Dietary Worksheet – Page 4

Macronutrient Calories per Day:

Calories from Carbs: = Cal_D __1917__ x 0.4 = Cal_C __767__ calories
Calories from Protein: = Cal_D __1917__ x 0.3 = Cal_P __575__ calories
Calories from Fat: = Cal_D __1917__ x 0.3 = Cal_F __575__ calories

Grams of Macronutrients per Day:

Grams of Carbohydrates = Cal_C __767__ ÷ 4 = __192__ grams
Grams of Protein   = Cal_P __575__ ÷ 4 = __144__ grams
Grams of Fat   = Cal_F __575__ ÷ 9 = __64__ grams

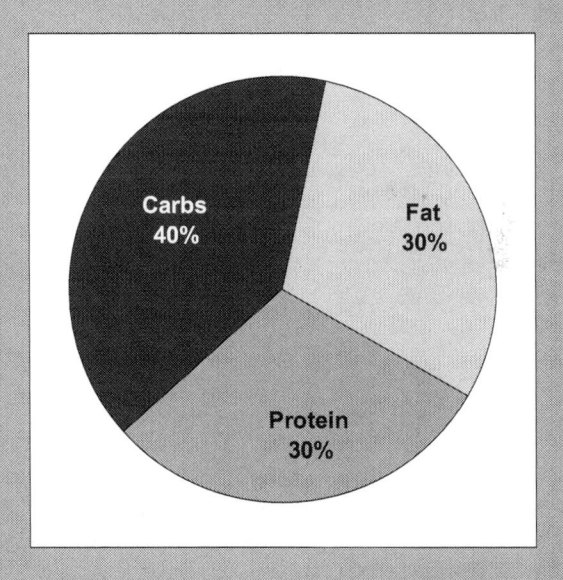

Carbs 40%
Fat 30%
Protein 30%

Chapter 15 - Whole Food

If you want to have a healthy diet and lifestyle there really is only one way to go and that is a whole food diet. There are lots of variations such as The Mediterranean Diet, the Caveman Diet and The Paleo Diet. These diets are all similar in that they promote eating exclusively whole foods.

Whole Food (hohl-food) *noun* 1. Food with little or no refining or processing and containing no artificial additives or preservatives. 2. A natural food and especially an unprocessed one such as a fruit or vegetable.

It's easy to tell if a food is a whole food. It is a single ingredient, not a bunch of unidentifiable chemicals thrown together in a lab. Whole foods often do not have a Nutritional Facts Label because it is easy to identify the ingredients; because there is only one. Non-whole foods have ingredients lists with lots of ingredients, including a bunch of items you may have never heard of.

For instance, here is the ingredients list from the label of a popular nutritional bar:

Ingredients: Chocolate Coating (Maltitol, Fractionated Palm Kernel Oil, Whey Protein Concentrate, Cocoa (processed with alkali), Calcium Carbonate, Naturals Flavors, Soy Lecithin, Sucralose), Hydrolyzed Collagen, Peanut Flour, Glycerin, Protein Blend (Whey Protein Hydrolysate, Whey Protein Isolate), Maltitol Syrup, Soy Crisps (Soy Protein Isolate, Tapioca Starch, Salt), Water, Peanuts, Peanut Oil, Sucrose, Soy Protein Isolate, Salt, Natural Flavor, Calcium Carbonate, Vitamin and Mineral Blend (Ascorbic Acid, d-Alpha Tocopheryl Acetate, Niacinamide, Tricalcium Phosphate, Zinc Oxide, Copper Gluconate, d-Calcium Pathothenate, Vitamin A Palmitate, Pyridoxine Hydrochloride, Thiamin, Riboflavin, Folic Acid, Biotin, Potassium Iodide, Cyanocobalamin), Sucralose, Soy Lecithin, Milk Protein Isolate, Almond Butter.

On the front label it says "Naturally Flavored" and "Eat Good, Look Great"

As you can clearly see, there is a big difference between "health food" and whole food. I'm no chemist, but that health food bar is not looking so healthy to me.

Now we look at the label of a bag of Planters Trail Mix.

Ingredients: Peanuts, Raisins, Dried Bananas, Sugar, Cashews, Dried Pineapple, Coconut Oil, Dried Cranberries, contains 2% or less of: Citric Acid, Peanut Oil, Sea Salt, Natural Flavor, Sulfur Dioxide added to preserve color.

In a strict sense this is not absolutely whole food, but the difference is clear. The first product was made by a chemist in a lab, the second product is just food. We like to joke that you can identify whole food by looking at the label... If it has a label, it's not whole food.

Whole food is close to the Earth and close to the farm. Let's take a look at some whole foods and their processed food counter parts.

Whole Food	Processed Food
Trail Mix	Nutrition Bar
Turkey Breast	Sliced Deli Turkey
Beef Tenderloin	Canned Ravioli
Corn on the Cob	Canned Corn
Fresh Tomatoes	Chunky Spaghetti Sauce
Natural Peanut Butter	Jarred Peanut Butter
Apples	Store Bought Apple Sauce
Bacon	Bacon Bits
Whole Milk	Sports Drink
Head of Lettuce	Bag of Lettuce
Bag of Whole Grain	Bag of Flour
Mushrooms	Canned Cream of Mushroom
Soy Beans	Soy Burgers
Black Beans	Black Bean Burger
Potatoes	French Fries

You can make all of the items on the right yourself, in your own kitchen, using only whole food. But chances are, if you buy them from a store or restaurant it will be loaded with additives and preservatives.

Law #25 -
Skip the Processed Food and stick to a Whole Food Diet.

Processed foods made in a laboratory, filled with additives and preservatives, processed flour and sugar, and countless chemicals are not healthy. If you want to live a long healthy life, skip the processed food.

Watch out for the Health Food bait and switch. Health food is not always so healthy.

Convenience Food

We talk about eating intentionally, planning out your meals and eating whole food; but how do you stick to that plan?

The goal is to think of food in an altogether different way. Don't eat because you're hungry or because you have a craving or because it is lunch time. Eat because you need to provide your body with specific nutrition at specific times, in order to maximize health. Like a pharmacist filling a prescription.

Looking back to Law #3, Meal Preparation is the biggest saboteur of a healthy diet. Your best intentions are not good enough. You must plan out your meals in advance.

What are you going to eat tomorrow? What is breakfast? What is lunch? What is dinner? What are your snacks between meals? What times do you need to eat? Are you balancing your macronutrients? Are you following the plan from your dietary worksheet? All these questions need to be answered well in advance of meal time.

Frozen Meals:

When it comes to frozen meals you can see by reading the labels those "healthy" frozen meals are not so healthy. Loaded with sugar, chemicals and who knows what; your frozen food options simply won't do.

Consider making your own frozen meals. A few plastic containers and lids go a long way. You can make 2 or 3 of your favorite dishes on the weekend, freeze them and eat them throughout the week.

Eating Out:

When it comes to eating out at restaurants it is often difficult to make healthy choices. Consider making a list of local restaurants and finding one or two menu items that meet your nutritional needs. Obviously most fast food and many other restaurants will not work for your new healthy lifestyle; but you'll find that many places will have one or two healthy selections.

It becomes a lot easier to eat out if you have already looked at the menu, went to the restaurant web page to read the Nutritional Facts page, and decided what you are going to eat, all before walking through the door.

Vegetarianism

I am not personally a vegetarian (today), but the lure of being a vegetarian is sometimes hard to resist once you understand the full reasoning behind it. I consider myself "Vegetarian Lite", meaning I do eat meat, but not too much.

Let's take a look at the reasons why some people are vegetarians. Once you are educated on the topic you can make the decision for yourself.

Political Vegetarian:

Some people do not eat meat because they consider it wrong to kill animals and eat their flesh. Other people have a problem with the way animals are raised in factory farms.

I will not discuss the politics and ethics behind eating meat; that topic is for a different book. However, I will say in no subtle way, the living conditions on factory farms are horrific. Watch a few YouTube videos on factory farms and you may never eat meat again.

Most vegetarians are not primarily interested in the politics and ethics of eating animals. They are more interested in the nutritional aspects of not eating animals. They correctly believe that you can live a more healthy life by avoiding meat and animal products.

The problem for most people is, even if you completely agree with the nutritional aspects of being a vegetarian or vegan (no animal products), vegetarianism can be very impractical. Being a true vegetarian takes some work and planning, but it may be worth the effort. You decide.

Saturated Fats:

Meat products are loaded with unwanted saturated fats. As you know from our discussion on fat as a macronutrient, saturated fat is not good for you. Eating saturated fat increases your risk for heart disease and stroke. Saturated fats and cholesterol will clog up your arteries and lead to life threatening blockages. Saturated fats contribute to inflammatory disorders and increase free radicals in your body.

Saturated fats are not preferred and should be avoided. However, as I like to say, everything in moderation. Eat saturated fat, just not too much. Skip the hamburger, the T-bone steak and the turkey drumstick and go for much leaner cuts of meat or poultry. If you are avoiding excess saturated fat, as you should be for a healthy diet, stick with filet and white meat poultry like chicken breasts.

Even with these lean cuts of meat, you want to keep it to a minimum by eating meat only a few times per week.

Food *Per 100 grams*	*Fat* *grams*	*Saturated* *grams*	*Mono* *grams*	*Poly* *grams*	*Cholesterol* *mg*
Hotdog	30.3	12.5	14.7	1.4	80
Hamburger	20	8.8	7.8	1	60
Bologna	22.7	7	9.7	3.5	25
Rabbit	10	3.2	2	1.9	80
Rib eye	6	2.9	2.6	0.2	62
Pork Loin	5.9	2.3	1	2.1	66
Roast Beef	5.7	1.4	2	0	55
Turkey Leg	3.6	1.3	0.8	0.9	40
Venison Loin	2.4	1.1	0.6	0.1	40
Beef Tenderloin	2.3	1	0.9	0.2	55
Chicken Leg	2.3	0.7	0.6	0.5	74
Turkey Breast	1.4	0.3	0.2	0.2	15
Chicken Breast	0.9	0.2	0.2	0.2	45

Source: FoodNutritionTable.com

Disease Prevention:

There is a popular belief among vegetarians that eating animal products causes disease in humans. The cause of the disease includes saturated fats, free radicals, pH imbalance, hormones, chemicals, etc.

The illnesses reportedly caused by meat consumption include cancer, heart disease, chronic inflammation, stomach and esophageal disease, infections like salmonella and many many more.

My use of the word "reportedly" might indicate that I don't have full buy-in to this concept. The truth is that overconsumption of animal products is a significant contributor to these diseases. However, it is only one of many environmental factors causing disease. Also, take note of the word "overconsumption". Everything in moderation. How much is too much?

While vegetarians set their "meat limit" to zero, I set mine just a little higher.

It is a widely held belief in the holistic medicine community and especially in the vegetarian community that cancer cannot thrive in an alkaline body. An acid pH level in the body is a magnet for cancer, disease and premature aging.

pH level varies from person to person depending on the things you choose to consume. Avoiding acidy animal products while eating more alkaline foods like vegetables helps you shift your pH level away from acidity and more toward alkalinity.

Read "The pH Miracle: Balance Your Diet, Reclaim Your Health" by Robert and Shelley Young, or any number of other books found on Amazon.com related to "pH balance and disease" for more information on how pH balance leads to disease prevention.

Toxic Factory Farms:

There are many vegetarians who have no problem eating meat, but do object to eating the meat available to Americans from modern factory farms. They will eat free range or private farm raised animal products, but altogether avoid animal products found in the grocery store or restaurants.

Why?

Animals raised on factory farms are given pesticides, growth hormones and antibiotics in large volumes to maximize meat production. As a result, these animals are extra fatty and filled with unnatural toxic chemicals which then get passed on to you. Stress hormones from living in these intense conditions end up in the food we eat.

Chickens are de-beaked to avoid excess pecking, while they are forced to exist inside overcrowded pens filled with their own squalor of droppings, feathers and other waste. Animals living their whole life around reeking open cesspools of excrement and waste.

Because of the horrific living conditions on these factory farms, animals are not healthy. They are slaughtered with festering wounds and any number of diseases. Don't worry too much because the diseased meat is cleaned with bleach and ammonia before you eat it.

The alternative of growing your own food is impractical for most of us, so we just skip the meat.

Intentional Eating:
Intentional eating means choosing the food you eat based on nutritional content instead of based on flavor or convenience. When you eat intentionally like a pharmacist filling a prescription, you are careful to always select food that meets your nutritional needs.

Many vegetarians are not so much avoiding meat, but intentionally eating things to satisfy their nutritional needs. Leaving meat out of your diet leaves room for eating more vegetables, nuts, seeds, etc.

While some vegetarians are all about eating intentionally, other vegetarians have a BAD diet. There are three common problems.

- Many vegetarians replace unhealthy meats with unhealthy carbohydrates which leads to just as many problems.

- Meats are particularly full of protein. Cutting out the meat can make it difficult for you to obtain the appropriate levels of protein. If you are going to skip the meat, you must be sure to get your protein from other sources such as whey, casein, pea protein, legumes, and high protein vegetables.

Remember that most plant proteins are incomplete. So it takes some extra effort to make sure you're eating the complimentary incomplete proteins in order to form the complete proteins your body needs.

- Processed food! Being a vegetarian is a lot of effort. Some vegetarians replace unhealthy meats with processed foods like soy burgers and "nutritional bars". Replacing meat for processed food is not a good exchange.

These are pretty compelling arguments for vegetarianism. You might be wondering how I can promote eating meat given these facts. I go back to "Everything in Moderation".

Chapter 16 - Reading Labels

You can't eat intentionally if you don't know what you are eating. If you are anything like most people in America, you shop and eat completely oblivious to the nutritional content of what you are eating. Your new healthy diet and lifestyle requires you to know exactly what you are eating. Not to figure out what you just ate, but to know what you are about to eat.

Whole Food:

We have discussed that most whole food does not have a Nutrition Facts Label, so you'll have to look it up on-line at a web page like FoodNutritionTable.com or use a smart phone application like MyFittnessPal. Both of these methods allow you to easily find and track the nutritional information about almost all whole foods.

Restaurants:

Lots of popular restaurants already have items indexed in MyFittnessPal. All you have to do is enter in the name of the restaurant and the item and you have a good chance of finding it in the application.

A better approach is to go to the restaurant web page. Most will have a nutritional facts page available on-line or a paper version in the store. Using this guide you can see exactly what you are eating. If the restaurant is not willing to provide you with the information you need to make a good choice, you need to eat someplace else. What are they hiding anyway?

Don't be afraid to make a special order or special modifications. Often you can take an unhealthy meal and make it healthy by removing the sauce and adding a vegetable. Ask for it grilled instead of fried. Trade out the french fries for a sweet potato.

Nutrition Facts Label:

Most packaged food in the grocery store has a special panel on the back called the Nutritional Facts Label. Between this label and the list of ingredients, you can make an educated decision if you should eat the food. The fact that the food is packaged to begin with is an indication that it is not part of a healthy diet, but the label can help you know for sure.

The Nutrition Facts Label is based on a generic person, not you. The Food and Drug Administration made it in 1968 considering a 2000 calorie daily diet. They have more recently updated the Recommended Daily Allowance for some of the vitamins and minerals.

Let's analyze the label and see what we can see.

Diet – Reading Labels

① Servings ➡

② Calories ➡

③ Fats ➡

④ Electrolytes ➡

⑤ Carbs ➡

⑥ Proteins ➡

⑦ Nutrients ➡

⑧ Footnote ➡

Nutrition Facts

Serving Size 1 oz (28g/about 28 nuts)
Servings Per Package 16

Amount Per Serving

Calories 170   Calories from Fat 140

	% Daily Value *
Total Fat 16g	24%
Saturated Fat 1g	6%
Trans Fat 0g	
Cholesterol 0mg	0%
Sodium 85mg	4%
Potassium 190mg	5%
Total Carbohydrate 5g	2%
Dietary Fiber 3g	11%
Sugars 1g	
Protein 6g	

Vitamin A 0%	•	Vitamin C 0%
Calcium 8%	•	Iron 6%
Vitamin E 35%	•	Magnesium 20%

* Percentage Daily Values are based on a 2,000 calorie diet. Your daily values may be higher or lower depending on your calorie needs:

	Calories	2,000	2,500
Total Fat	Less than	65g	80g
Sat. Fat	Less than	20g	25g
Cholesterol	Less than	300mg	300mg
Sodium	Less than	2,400mg	2,400mg
Potassium		3,500mg	3,500mg
Total Carbohydrate		300g	375g
Dietary Fiber		25g	30g

Diet – Reading Labels

① Servings:

It is very important to observe the serving size and servings per container. Often you think your item is a single serving, but they sneak in extra calories by saying 2.5 servings per container. Watch out for their tricks!

② Calories:

Not all calories are created equal. High quality matters a lot more than low calorie. Make sure you are eating the right food before you ever worry about calories.

Remember fat has lots of calories but makes you feel full and satisfied. Stay within your calorie budget according to your plan.

③ Fats:

You need fat! Eat it. Love it. But remember to go easy on the bad Saturated Fat and completely avoid toxic Trans Fat. Be careful not to go crazy on the Cholesterol.

④ Electrolytes:

Sodium and Potassium are very important electrolytes, critical to neurological function. Remember to increase your electrolytes to replenish those lost during exercise. But, keep your sodium intake under control and don't go overboard. 2,000 mg per day is more or less a good limit, depending on your activity and climate.

⑤ Carbohydrates:

Refer to your Dietary Worksheet to see how many grams of carbs you should eat per day. Remember to skip items high in sugar to avoid the insulin roller coaster. Look for items high in healthy fiber.

⑥ Proteins:

Refer to your Dietary Worksheet to see how many proteins you should eat per day. Sometimes it is tough to get 30% of your calories from protein, so you will need to seek them out.

⑦ Nutrients:

Make sure you are getting plenty of micronutrients in your diet. You may need to take quality supplements to get these up to appropriate levels.

⑧ Footnote:

The Footnote is the same on every label. It is the Food and Drug Administration's recommendation for the American diet. These recommendations are very old and not specific to your needs. Use the Dietary Worksheet to calculate your specific needs.

Chapter 17 - The Magic Formula Diet

Everybody is looking for the magic pill or the magic bullet to make their weight loss easy. Unfortunately, there is no "one thing". Weight loss and having a healthy diet and lifestyle is a major lifestyle change for most people. You must get your head wrapped around the idea that you are going to have to start doing things differently for the rest of your life.

What works for living and eating healthy is a permanent change; conscious lifestyle changes of eating and exercising intentionally. I provide for you my Magic Formula Diet. It is a comprehensive plan designed for you to be healthy and reach your optimal weight.

Calories

Many diets focus on calories, but not this one. Why? Because not all calories are the same. Focus on eating the right food first. Only then do calories start to matter.

Calories are the energy stored in the food you eat. If you consume more energy than you use, it gets stored as fat. Consider the fact that your current weight and fat storage is the net sum of everything you have ever eaten and every activity you've ever done. Remember, when you eat some bad food "this will go on your permanent record".

A pound of fat is around 3500 calories, so to lose one pound you are going to need to have a deficiency of 3500 calories. It is best if you spread that out over a long period of time. And remember, if your calorie intake is too low, your body will go into starvation mode.

Bottom line for calories:

- Calories are secondary behind food quality.
- Use the Dietary Worksheet to calculate your needs.

Metabolic Recovery Days

All this calorie deficiency stuff will destroy your metabolism if you go too long. You need to send your body the right message: There is plenty of food, no need to store fat energy for later.

Diet – The Magic Formula Diet

Once per week, have a metabolic recovery day when you eat a normal (non-deficient) calorie count, or maybe a little extra. You can see in the Dietary Worksheet what your BMR is. Make sure you eat at least that many calories (adjusted up for exercise) on your recovery day.

- Send your body the right message. There is plenty of food.

Eat Often

You need to keep your campfire burning. Don't skip meals and eat plenty of snacks to keep your metabolism running strong all day and night. These snacks are critical for timing your meals and exercise. An orange at 4:00 PM enables you to exercise at 6:00 PM before dinner.

- Eat breakfast immediately after you wake.
- Eat 6 or more times per day (every 3 to 4 hours).
- Eat healthy snacks between small meals.
- Never allow yourself to get overly hungry.
- Don't eat for two hours before bed. (a light snack is ok)

Balanced Macronutrients

You must balance your macronutrients for every meal and every day. You need fat for energy and to feel full. Fiber and energy from carbohydrates are fundamental to your diet. Proteins are often neglected or supplemented with poor quality supplements. Do not let common misconceptions stop you from getting the right amount of each macronutrient.

- Your daily calories should be 40% Carb, 30% Fat and 30% Protein.
- Use the Dietary Worksheet to calculate your macronutrient needs.
- Avoid the bad fats (saturated fat) and the toxic fats (trans fat).
- Seek out the healthy Omega 3, mono and poly unsaturated fats.

- Avoid high sugar carbs like HFCS and The White Menace flour and sugar.
- Look for carbs with lots of fiber.
- Avoid the insulin roller coaster by skipping high glycemic load foods and meals.

Whole Foods

You must eat primarily whole foods to maintain a healthy lifestyle. Read the ingredients, if it doesn't sound like "food", do not eat it. Eat unrefined, unprocessed whole foods with no artificial additives or preservatives. Eat natural food which is close to the ground and close to the farm.

Avoid eating processed food. The more processed, the worse it is for you. Keep in mind that the food industry's goal is to make money, not to serve you healthy food. We crave sugar, fat and salt. They are just providing the supply to our demand for cheap, fast and easy food that tastes good.

Change the paradigm and demand high quality whole food instead of the processed food.

Think about one of these mega-food companies. They buy the whole food from the farms. They cut it up, cook it, process it, add in trans fat, salt, MSG, and millions of tons of chemicals. They package it and put it in a pretty box. Then they have to label it so you can try to figure out what the heck you are actually eating. Next they ship it across the country or across the world, where we then pop it into our microwave ovens and eat it.

Cut out the middle man. Get the whole food and eat that instead.

- Avoid forever highly processed foods. Never eat another hotdog, bologna sandwich, chicken nugget or can of ravioli.
- Eat whole foods.
- Eat foods close to the earth and close to the farm.
- Read the ingredients; if it doesn't sound like food, it's not.
- Go easy on the convenience food like frozen meals and restaurants.

Veggie Lite

Meats and poultry offer a great source of protein and can be a part of a healthy diet. But too much can be a bad thing. Between the saturated fats and the slipping quality of the American food source, animal products ain't what they used to be.

Keep your pH balance alkaline, and your arteries free from clogging cholesterol by cutting back on the meat.

- Limit only one serving of lean tenderloin per week.
- Eat mostly fish and white meat poultry for your meat source.
- Search for quality sources for animal products (good luck).
- Supplement with quality protein sources like whey, casein, and natural plant and nut proteins.

Avoid Too Much Soy Protein

Avoiding soy protein was the key to unlocking my personal fat loss. This omnipresent food additive is commonly used as a protein filler in much of the processed foods we eat. It is cheap and easy for food companies to load us up on soy instead of other quality protein sources; therefore we eat way too much.

I do not recommend avoiding soy lecithin or soy oil, just soy protein. Read your labels. If soy protein or soy protein isolate is listed within the first 3 or 4 items, you might want to take a pass.

- Soy protein will lower your free testosterone.
- Soy protein will increase your estrogen.
- Soy protein will cause several different hormone imbalances that will each make you gain weight and retain fat.

I'm not recommending truly removing soy protein from your diet. However, you should understand the hormonal effects of soy and keep it to a reasonable limit in your diet.

Drink Water

Drink lots and lots of water. Drink water when you wake up in the morning. Drink water with every meal. Drink several glasses of water between meals. Drink water in the middle of the night. Drink, drink, drink.

Water will flush your system and help remove toxins. It has a thermogenic effect. It will raise your metabolism and help you burn fat. It will do the dishes and wash the laundry. (Okay, maybe I got a little carried away)

Optimally you will exclude all other beverages and drink exclusively water. Whatever you do, skip the high sugar drinks and the artificially sweetened drinks.

- Drink lots of water, all day, every day.
- Don't drink calories

Take Supplements

My philosophy is to eat nutritious whole food for your main source of nutrients, then fill in the gaps with supplements. Which supplements do you need? Good question.

There are so many great supplements available to you, it's hard not to go crazy taking them all. This is another topic that can be a whole book all on its own. I suggest you take a look at all these supplements and figure out which are right for you.

Omega 3:

If you are not eating fish every day, you may be very low on the healthy fatty acid Omega 3. Actually, no matter what you're eating, it is difficult to get as much as you need. Consider using flaxseed oil or a fish oil supplement to boost your level. Not all fish oil is created equal. High quality dark fish oil is much better than flaxseed or white fish oil.

Superfruits:

Many foods such as acai berry, lyceum berry, maqui berry, noni-fruit and many more are called super-fruits. These foods will boost your energy and charge your immune system with antioxidants and anti-inflammatory properties.

Thermogenics:

Although there are thermogenic foods, it may be much easier to boost your metabolism through thermogenic supplements.

- Garlic
- Alpha Lipoic Acid
- Green Tea Extract
- Ginger

Vitamins and Minerals:

Vitamins A, B Complex, C, D, E and minerals such as iron, magnesium, calcium and others are micronutrients required for healthy living. You must consume these through eating lots of healthy whole foods, or supplements.

You may find that it is very difficult to eat all of the micronutrients you need. Supplements are a good alternative.

You should know that vitamin D is not actually a vitamin, but a hormone. You need plenty of sunlight in order to produce appropriate levels of vitamin D, otherwise you'll need a supplement.

Meal Replacement Shakes

Meal replacement shakes are a great way to get high nutritional content in a small calorie package. A quick shake for breakfast or as a snack can keep you satisfied for hours.

Be careful, you must choose a high quality meal replacement shake. Skip the soy protein and look for something healthy like pea protein or a scientifically balanced protein blend. Don't go overboard, only have meal replacement shakes for one or two of your six meals.

A protein shake is great for exercise recovery, but a meal replacement shake should have a healthy mix of macronutrients. Make sure it has plenty of carbs.

Exercise Daily

You should exercise 6 days per week. Strength training several days and cardio training several days.

This workout program should be tailored to your own special needs. Walking and pool activities are great for people who are unable to do more strenuous activity. The point is to get your heart rate elevated. Strength training can be heavy weight or light weight depending on your abilities, but it is important to tone up your muscles and increase your lean body mass.

Vigorous exercise for long durations is great for getting fit, <u>but may work against you for weight loss goals</u>.
- Cardio: walking, swimming, running, etc. several times per week.
- Strength training to increase your LBM, do it a few times per week.

Why We Plateau and How to Break It.

The plateau is a big problem for many dieters. You diet and starve yourself only to stay the same weight for weeks. Sometimes it seems like you are working so hard but not making any progress. How do you break the plateau?

Too much exercise:

> Doing too much cardio will send your body the wrong messages. You end up being extra hungry and eating all day. Skip the run and go for a walk for better results.

Too much cheating:

> A little extra here and there can destroy your diet. If you are on a plateau, make sure you are logging every bite. If you eat out too much, you might be cheating and not even know it.

Not Serious about it:

> I always found it so insulting that some people think I'm not serious about diet and exercise just because I was not losing weight. The big misconception is that all you have to do is eat less and exercise more and you will lose weight. Not true.

> With that said. If you are not serious about losing fat, if you are not following the laws, you need to rethink your priorities and goals.

Campfire burning out:
> Just because you are on a diet does not mean you should skip meals. Eat to lose. 5 or 6 meals per day are best. <u>Never ever skip breakfast</u>.

Losing LBM:
> When you diet to lose weight, you will likely lose fat and muscle. Losing LBM will lower your metabolism. Strength training will help.

Ice Age Metabolism:
> When you diet too much and eat too few calories for too long, your metabolism will plummet. You need lots of metabolic recovery days to break the cycle. Eat lots of calories of healthy whole foods, especially unsaturated fats like avocados and nuts.

You might have a food allergy or sensitivity:
> There is nothing wrong with eating gluten, unless you have a sensitivity to it. Celiac Disease can cause all kinds of dietary problems. Give up wheat for a week or two to see if you feel better.
>
> Some people are more sensitive to the effects of soy than others. Soy doesn't make everybody fat, but it could be making you fat.
>
> Consider getting a food allergy test to see if you have other problems.

Water:
> Not having enough water, particularly ice-water, is a non-starter for your healthy diet. You simply can't be healthy without drinking enough water.

Eating out too much:
> You know the problems with restaurant food. When you are not in control of the ingredients and the portions, all bets are off. Prepare your own foods for best results.

Exercise

Are you a Couch Potato? People who sit on the couch all day eating potato chips and drinking soda filled with HFCS will get fat, get sick and die. You need to get plenty of exercise to live a healthy lifestyle.

Everybody's exercise needs are different. You'll have to consider your own personal goals in order to determine what types of exercise you need. With that said, just about everybody needs some form of strength training and some sort of cardio.

If you do not exercise, you're probably thinking "Oh no, that sounds terrible. I'm tired and busy, and the last thing I want to do is exercise." I have great news for you... Exercise makes you feel great! And it is totally addictive!

When you exercise you get a brain chemical reward of serotonin and dopamine. After exercise you'll feel tired and sore, but you'll still feel great. That euphoria will keep you coming back for more.

Strength Training

Strength training is more than some muscle heads pumping iron at the gym; it is great for people who are twenty two to one hundred two. It is important to develop strong muscles and a healthy Lean Body Mass. Being strong will help you have a great metabolism and it will keep you looking and feeling young.

Cardio

Cardio or Cardiovascular Training will burn calories and fat and promote healthy heart and lung function. When you do lots of cardio your heart and lungs will get very strong, which helps in all aspects of your life. Do you get a little winded walking up a flight of stairs? It might be time to work on that cardio.

Chapter 18 - Strength Training

Strength training really is important for just about every body. Men, women, old and young, all need to have a healthy amount of muscle mass, best achieved by strength training.

I'm not going to talk about weight lifting technique and methodology. The strength training requirements for a petite 82 year old woman and an obese 43 year old man are totally different. Both require just the right strength training routine tailored to their own specific personal needs.

So instead of talking about how to strength train, we will discuss the benefits of strength training and how to get started right.

Looking back at the equation for calculating your Basal Metabolic Rate:

$$BMR = LBM \times 13.8$$

That means for every pound of Lean Body Mass you will burn about 13.8 calories. Therefore, the more muscle mass you have the more calories you will burn. Doing strength training will really boost your metabolism and help you burn more calories than ever.

Considering Percentage Body Fat, we discussed healthy ratios of fat and muscle. In general you want to minimize your fat and maximize your muscle.

Healthy Body Fat for Men
- Ages 20-39: 8% to 19%
- Ages 40-59: 11% to 21%
- Ages 60+ : 13% to 24%

Healthy Body Fat for Women
- Ages 20-39: 21% to 32%
- Ages 40-59: 23% to 33%
- Ages 60+ : 24% to 35%

Converting fat mass to muscle mass, by doing strength training will help you achieve a healthy Body Fat Percentage. This will lead to better cardiac health and a longer life.

Elderly, frail, skinny fat and just plain skinny body types in particular need to gain more muscle mass in order to reach optimal health. These folks need a special kind of strength training starting with light resistance training.

Using your own body weight, stretch bands, wrist and ankle weights, small dumbbells or light kettle bells are all great for starting your training. Beginning weight trainers can start with simple squats or lunges, wall pushups and other exercises. You can find lots of strength training ideas on-line by searching for "Beginning Strength Training". However, the best way to get started is by working with a personal trainer to teach you the basics.

There are several at home videos that will help you with strength training basics. I like Beach Body's Power 90 for beginners and P90X for the more advanced folks. But there are lots of other choices; some are available for free on-line. Search for "strength training video" in Google or YouTube to see your options.

For most people who are in reasonable health, I recommend you join a gym, get a personal trainer and do strength training three times per week. Consider two upper body and one lower body weight lifting sessions per week.

You ladies don't need to worry about getting "Big and Bulky" because that is simply not going to happen. Instead, you will develop healthy muscle tone, and start burning off extra fat.

For the fellas, start off light and work your way up. It's not a competition, so don't hurt yourself!

Warning: If you do strength training exercises wrong you can and will hurt yourself. Be careful and get a personal instruction to avoid injury. Seriously!

Chapter 19 - Cardio

Cardio (kär-dē-ō) *noun* 1. Exercise intended to temporarily raise your heart rate to 50% or more of maximum heart rate, for some extended duration (typically 20 minutes or more).

Your body needs cardio exercise in order to stay healthy. More so, the absence of cardio exercise will make you fat and lazy, and will lead to having a weak heart, weak lungs and a generally unhealthy body. Get off your butt and do some cardio.

Just like with strength training, everybody's cardio exercise needs are going to be different. Depending on your condition, you'll need to choose an exercise that is right for you. You should definitely get checked out by a doctor before you start a new cardio regimen. If you haven't had one in a while, make sure you get a full checkup and talk to your doctor about your plans.

I realize this sounds like a standard "cover your butt" disclaimer which may be ignored or not taken seriously, however it is not. I am very serious. Go get a checkup before you start.

When I first started training for triathlon I got a full checkup, EKG, Stress Test with Echo, and a Pulmonary Function Test (because of my asthma). I was having some chest pain during exercise, but it turned out to be respiratory. The cold dry winter air was hurting my lungs. I wear a mask in the winter to help with that now.

Once you have approval from your doctor, it's time to get started. For beginners and people working on losing weight, I recommend 45 minutes of light cardio, four times per week. For more experienced people, I recommend 45 minutes of HIIT, five times per week.

Cardio vs. HIIT
For many years old fashioned cardio training was recommended, but now HIIT is the new method of choice. HIIT stands for High Intensity Interval Training. With normal cardio workouts you would get your heart rate up and keep it there for a while. With interval training you would work hard and then take a break, repeatedly.

Exercise – Cardio

For example, a jogger doing cardio may run three 10 minute miles for 30 minutes at 75% heart rate. Whereas an interval trainer might do 10-20-30's, which is sprinting for 10 seconds, jogging for 20 seconds and walking for 30 seconds.

With High Intensity Interval Training you would reverse it to 30-20-10, sprint for 30 seconds, jog for 20 seconds, walk for 10 seconds.

Here is a graph showing traditional cardio where the jogger gets his heart rate up to 75% and keeps it there for a while.

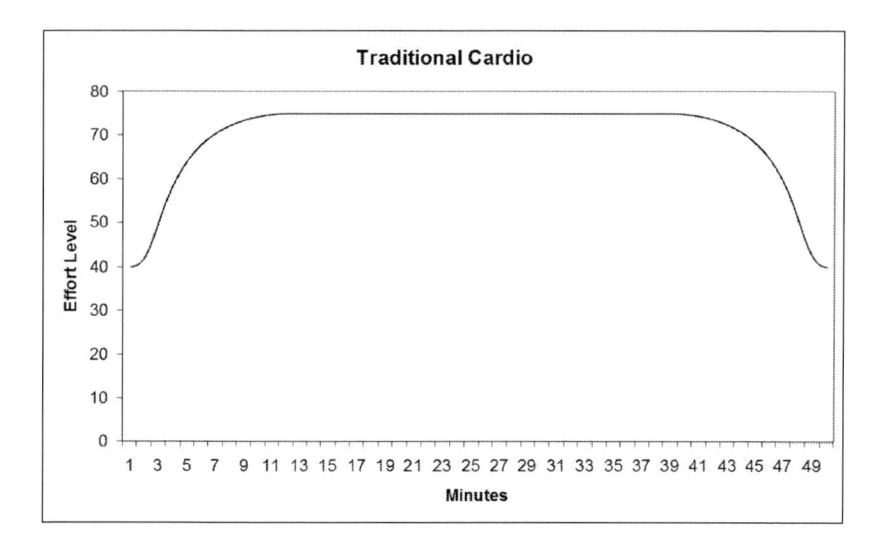

Exercise – Cardio

With interval training you can see the heart rate going up and down with short intervals of high exertion and longer intervals of lower exertion.

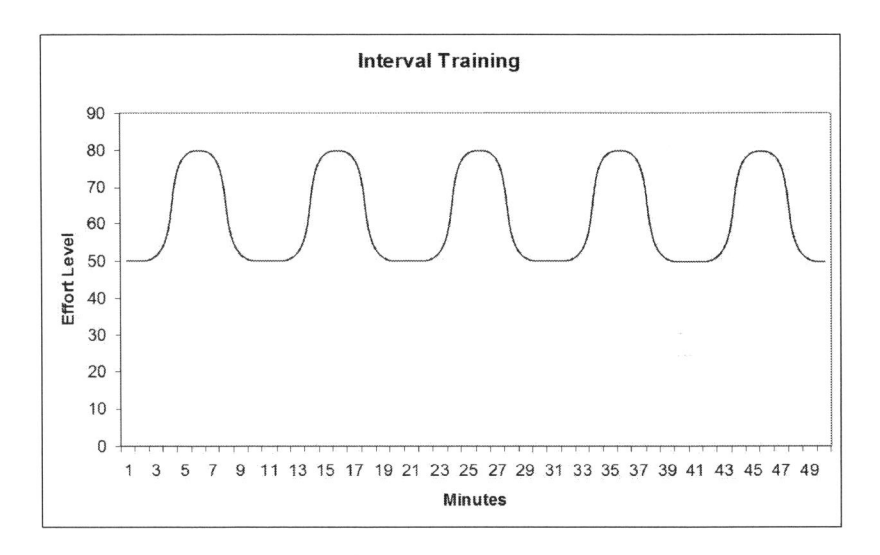

With High Intensity Interval Training you can see that the heart rate has higher highs, lower lows and the intense intervals last longer.

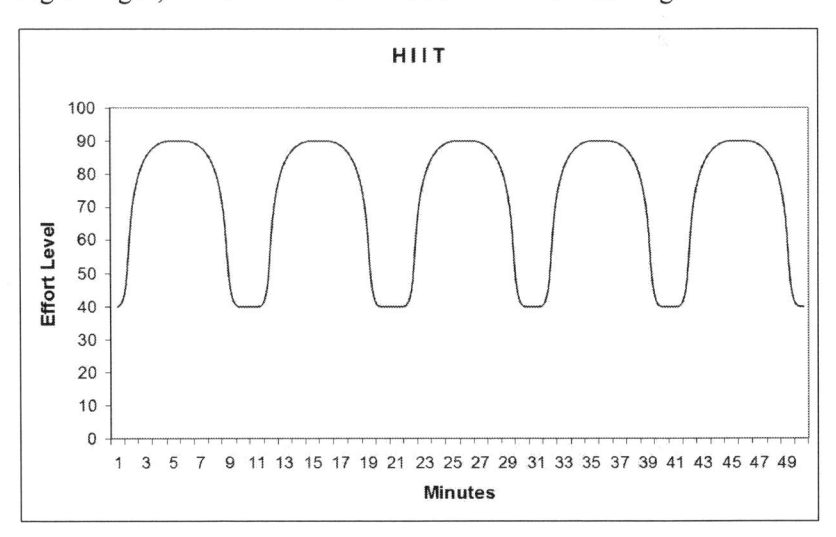

This next graph shows all three overlaid on top of each other so you can really compare the difference. HIIT is much more intense than the others.

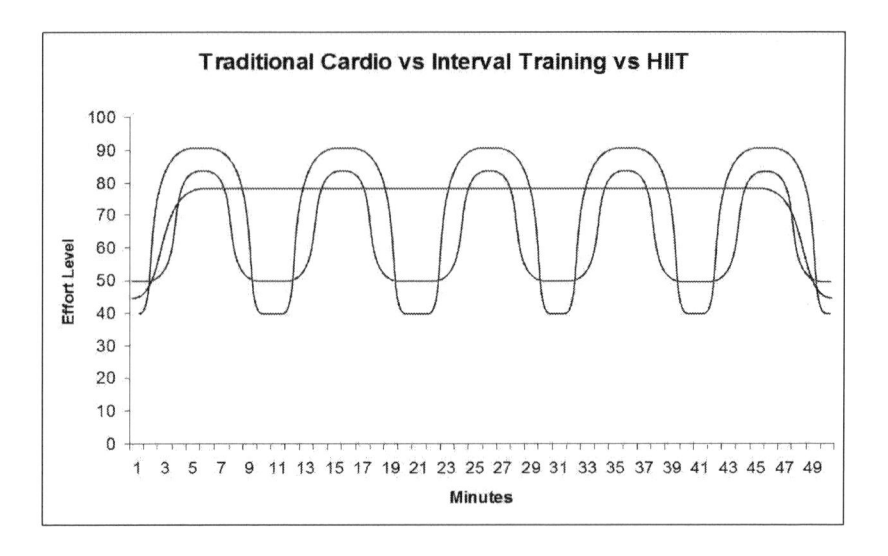

Traditional Cardio vs Interval Training vs HIIT

You can choose any combination cardio activity and method that works for you, your fitness level and goals. Remember, if you are intending to lose weight, you need to stay away from heavy cardio. I've already beat that drum, so I'm not getting into those details again.

Exercise – Cardio

Here is a list of ideas for you.

- Walking
- Hiking
- Cycling
- Hill Climbing
- Running
- Rollerblading
- Rowing
- Skiing
- Dancing
- Triathlon

- Treadmill
- Stair Climbing
- Stationary Bike
- Elliptical
- Swimming
- Water Aerobics
- Water Jogging
- Zumba
- Turbokick
- Mud & Obstacle Racing

- Jumping Jacks
- Jump Rope
- Squat Thrusts
- Kettlebells
- Step Aerobics
- Tennis
- Racquetball
- Basketball
- Martial Arts
- Boxing

Popular Workout Videos

- Insanity
- Brazil Butt Lift
- Biggest Loser Workout

- T25
- Sweatin' to the Oldies
- Power 90

- 30-Day Shred
- Hip Hop Abs
- Turbo Jam

Think about your car or any other mechanical device you own. The more you use it, the more worn out it gets. Most things get worn out from overuse. The human body, on the other hand, is a little different. The more you use your body, the stronger it gets.

When you do strenuous activities like strength training or cardio, your body responds by getting stronger and healthier. Cardio exercise will have fantastic effects on your entire cardiovascular system, your respiratory system, and your musculoskeletal system. The endorphin release from exercise will keep you coming back for more. Plus, you will burn calories and fat whenever you do aerobic exercise.

Aerobic vs. Anaerobic Training

When doing cardio, your body operates in two general modes; aerobic and anaerobic. While in the aerobic mode you are primarily using fat and oxygen as fuel. In this mode you are burning fat. In anaerobic mode your muscles are using primarily glycogen (sugar) stored in the muscles.

The big difference is that you have a seemingly endless supply of energy for aerobic exercise, but a very limited amount of energy stored for anaerobic exercise. For example, you may have enough fat storage to run for 30 days, but enough glycogen to run in the anaerobic mode for an hour or two.

Of course you do not simply switch back and forth between the two modes. At low heart rates you are primarily aerobic, while at high heart rates you are primarily anaerobic.

Considering this, during traditional cardio you spend a while just below or just above the anaerobic threshold; while interval training takes you well above and well below the anaerobic threshold.

If the goal is to lose fat, you want to keep your heart rate low and stay in the aerobic mode. However, if your goal is to improve fitness, you want to do HIIT. There are entire books dedicated to this topic, but I'm just scratching the surface.

One way to know you are in the aerobic zone is your ability to talk. If you can carry on a conversation, your heart rate is low and you are primarily aerobic. If you are working too hard to talk, you are primarily anaerobic.

I recommend heart rate zone training. Heart rate zones 1 and 2 are aerobic, while heart rate zone 4 is anaerobic.

Heart Rate Zones

It is important to monitor your heart rate, which is why I wear a heart rate monitor with alarms. If my heart rate drops too low or goes too high, my Heart Rate Monitor starts to beep indicating I'm out of my heart rate zone.

Training at too high a heart rate can be counterproductive, while training at too low a heart rate can be a waste of time. Know what heart rate zone you require to meet your fitness goals, set the alarms on your heart rate monitor and stick to the plan.

It's easy to get carried away with the exercise and push too hard. But it is much better for your health and fitness goals to stick to the plan; whatever your plan happens to be.

We'll get back to this in a minute.

Max Heart Rate

To calculate your heart rate zones you first need to start with your max heart rate. Your max heart rate is the highest possible heart rate you can achieve doing a specific activity, usually found during a stress test at a doctor's office or with trained fitness testing professional. Essentially, you run on a treadmill while they watch your heart rate climb. When it stops climbing, you've reached your maximum heart rate.

You may be thinking the obvious thought... You don't need a doctor to take that measurement. The problem is when you get your heart rate up to the maximum, you risk serious cardiac complications such as cardiac arrhythmia like Ventricular Fibrillation. Unless a trained medical professional is around when this happens, you pretty much always die. **Death is counterproductive to reaching your fitness goals, but it is great for weight loss.**

With that said, most people just use the formula to approximate your max heart rate.

$$\text{Max Heart Rate} = 220 - \text{age}$$

Using this formula, my MaxHR is 180, but using measurements it comes out a little higher. As mentioned, your max heart rate varies depending on the activity. My max heart rate for running is 188 Beats per Minute. For cycling it is 182 BPM. For racquetball, it is 191 BPM.

Back to Heart Rate Zones.

Zone 1: 60% - 69% of MaxHR (Aerobic- Light exercise like brisk walking)

Zone 2: 70% - 85% of MaxHR (Aerobic- Medium exercise like cycling)

Zone 3: 86% - 89% of MaxHR (Anaerobic Threshold)

Zone 4: 90% - 95% of MaxHR (Anaerobic– Heavy exercise like sprinting)

You may have noticed these numbers correspond to the numbers from the Dietary Worksheet. When you were calculating how much time you spend exercising, you did it by calculating each zone.

If you recall, we use that information to calculate how many calories you use during exercise in order to find your total daily calorie intake. We can make those calculations because the calories burned during activity is very predictable based on your stats combined with your heart rate. Let's take a look.

Calculating Calories Based on Heart Rate

In order to calculate calories burned, use a heart rate monitor to find your average heart rate in beats per minute (HR) and duration of exercise in minutes (T). Those numbers along with your weight in pounds (W) and your age in years (A) go into the following formula.

Men:
$$Cal = \frac{[(A \times 0.2017) + (W \times 0.09036) + (HR \times 0.6309) - 55.0969\,] \times T}{4.184}$$

Women:
$$Cal = \frac{[(A \times 0.074) + (W \times 0.05741) + (HR \times 0.4472) - 20.4022\,] \times T}{4.184}$$

This formula found and used in the Dietary Worksheet within this book.

Law #26 -
Get plenty of exercise; both cardio and strength training.

Chapter 20 - Summary

I noticed a great post from Rob Maxwell, a fitness guru, coach and proprietor of Maxwell's Fitness Programs in Port Orlando, Florida. His post really summarized everything I'm telling you.

We'll call this Maxwell's Equation.

Successful Healthy Lifestyle	Unsuccessful Habits
Here is what we know our successful clients have done to lose weight:	We saw what people who did not reach their goal were doing or not doing:
1. Cardio 5-6 days per week	1. Cardio was inconsistent
2. Strength Training with <u>intensity</u> 3 days per week.	2. Strength training was weak, going through the motions, no intensity
3. Kept a food diary	3. Did not keep a food journal
4. Eat 4-6 times per day	4. Skipped breakfast & other meals
5. Did not drink alcohol	5. Drank alcohol
6. Got plenty of sleep	6. Did not get enough rest
7. Stayed Hydrated	7. Did not drink enough water
8. Worked out when they traveled	8. Did not ask questions
9. Asked for feedback regarding diet	9. Ate biggest meal at night
10. Set goals	10. Did not set goals

Law #27 -
Consistency is King. You can always find an excuse.

If you are looking for an excuse, you will always find one.

"I'm too busy today" "Nobody can watch the baby" "I had to work late"

There truly is always something that wants to get in the way of your healthy lifestyle. The secret is to let health be a high priority in your life. Look for a reason to stick to your plan, not an excuse to skip out. If you do not stick to your plan you will not get the results you want.

Summary

Law #1 - You cannot have good health unless good health is a priority.

If you want to have a healthy lifestyle, you're going to need to make it a priority in your life. Reaching and maintaining a healthy weight, eating wholesome nutritious food, and getting healthy exercise all need to be high on your priorities list.

Law #2 - Write Down Your Goals.

Writing down your goals is the first step toward reaching your goals. If you want to have a healthy lifestyle, you're going to first need to set some healthy lifestyle goals.

Law #3 - Schedule It! Put it on the calendar.

Healthy lifestyle doesn't just fit into your day. You need to schedule it, and then plan around it. With work, family, and everything else in our hectic lives, eating right and exercise does not happen by accident. You're going to need to schedule it in.

Law #4 - Meal Preparation is the Biggest Saboteur of a Healthy Lifestyle.

If you plan to swing by the drive through on the way to your destination, don't expect to be healthy. You need to plan out your meals in advance. Failing to plan is planning to fail.

Law #5 - You Can't Manage What You Don't Measure.

Logging your meals and exercise will go a long way toward helping you reach your goals. It will keep you accountable and show you where you need work.

Law #6 - Will power alone cannot overcome your desire to eat.

I sometimes think I just have no self-control. But the truth is that self-control just isn't enough. To live a healthy lifestyle you first need to control your body and brain chemistry.

Law #7 - The Insulin Rollercoaster, nobody rides for free!

High glycemic load meals will mess with your blood sugar. You need to control your carbohydrate intake in order to control your body chemistry. Go easy on the sugar, avoid the White Menace and HFCS.

Law #8 - You must control your body chemistry to control your appetite.

Dopamine, Serotonin, Cortisol, and Insulin all drive our desire to eat. Control these chemicals and you'll be able to reign in your appetite.

Summary

Law #9 - You are in complete control of your metabolism.

Your metabolism is not something assigned to you at birth. It is something you create over a lifetime of habits, both good and bad. Don't blame your genetics, blame your behavior. If you want a healthy metabolism, you're going to have to maintain healthy diet and exercise.

Law #10 - Breakfast really is the most important meal of the day.

Your body is like a campfire; you need to feed the flame with fuel. Your metabolism shuts down when you sleep. If you want to turn it back on, you'll need to break your fast with breakfast.

Law #11 - Eat a healthy snack or meal every 3 to 4 hours.

Don't let your campfire burn out. Keep the flame burning by adding fuel to the fire all day. Small healthy snacks spread out over the day are best for a healthy metabolism.

Law #12 - Your body will cling to fat when in starvation mode.

Don't expect to lose weight if you're in starvation mode. Depriving yourself calories day after day after day will cause you to have a greatly impaired metabolism.

Law #13 - Dieting will eat up your muscles.

It's hard to lose fat without losing muscle. When you have a calorie deficiency, your metabolism starts burning tissue as fuel. You want it to burn fat, but it wants to burn muscle. Weight training will help mitigate your loss.

Law #14 - Muscle Mass burns calories.

The higher your Lean Body Mass the greater your Basal Metabolic Rate. Pack on the muscle for automatic fat loss.

Law #15 - Simply Eating Less & Exercising More does not work.

Dieting is often counterproductive because you're sending your body the wrong message. Unfortunately, you need to trick your body into doing what you want.

Law #16 - To lose weight, you must send your body the right messages.

You need to send your brain and body the right messages. If you are constantly telling your body that there is a food shortage it will think you're living in an ice-age.

Law #17 - Permanent weight loss requires a permanent lifestyle change.

If you're looking to go on a diet, lose some weight, and then get back to your old lifestyle, don't even bother! You need to give up certain toxic foods forever. Chicken nuggets and hot dogs are no longer on the menu. Lifestyle change is permanent.

Law #18 - Don't Drink Calories! Avoid high sugar drinks.

It will be tough for you to stick to your new healthy lifestyle if you are drinking too many calories. Don't drink calories, drink water.

Law #19 - Drink Water. Drink 1/2 Oz for every pound of body mass.

Chances are, you don't drink nearly enough water. You need it for a healthy life. You can't lose weight without drinking more water.

Law #20 - You must eat intentionally to have a healthy diet & lifestyle.

Food is a drug. Are you a user or an abuser? Don't think of food as a treat or a reward. Food is supposed to be nutrition. Eat intentionally in order to consume the nutrients your body needs.

Law #21 - You must ignore all the diet misinformation.

There's an awful lot of garbage information floating around out there. Learn to cut through the BS, urban legends, old wives tales, and misinformation to find the healthy lifestyle fact and fiction.

Law #22 - You must have a balanced diet. Balance your macronutrients.

You should be eating 40% carbohydrates, 30% protein, and 30% fat for every meal, every day. Balancing your macronutrients is an important step toward living your new healthy lifestyle.

Law #23 - Your calories should be 40% Carb, 30% Protein & 30% Fat.

Um... I think I just said that. Too late to call it 26 Laws.

Law #24 - A healthy diet has a low glycemic load.

You can eat sugar and lots of carbohydrates, but adding fiber will keep you out of trouble. Orange juice will spike your blood sugar, but an orange will provide healthy nutrition. The difference is fiber. Fiber will slow the metabolizing of sugars into the blood and help keep your body chemistry in check.

Law #25 - Skip the Processed Food and stick to a Whole Food Diet.

Whole Food is the key! Quit eating crappy processed food and stick to nutritious farm food. Read your labels. If you can't figure out what it is, you shouldn't be eating it.

Law #26 - Get plenty of exercise; both cardio and strength training.

You can't have a healthy lifestyle and longevity sitting on the couch. Get up and get some exercise. You'll start to love it, I promise.

Law #27 – Consistency is King. You can always find an excuse.

Being healthy, eating right, and getting plenty of exercise are life long lifestyle choices. I know life is hectic. I know there are always other priorities in your life. But you need to make nutrition and regular exercise part of your life or else you will pay the price.

Obesity is an epidemic in America. Don't be a statistic!

Chapter 21 - Reading List

If you are anything like me, you can't get enough good information on this topic of healthy living through diet and exercise. I've provided a list of my personal favorite books for you to read. I don't necessarily agree with everything in these books, but I know that the vast majority of the information is good and useful. Enjoy.

UltraMetabolism – *Mark Hyman, M.D.*
The Simple Plan for Automatic Weight Loss

> "For many, losing weight is a never-ending struggle -- especially since our bodies are designed to keep weight on at all costs; it's a matter of survival. But a medical revolution is under way, showing us how to work with our bodies instead of against them to ignite the natural fat-burning furnaces that lie dormant within us. Drawing on the cutting-edge science of nutrigenomics -- how food talks to our genes -- Dr. Mark Hyman has created a way of losing weight by eating the right foods, which in turn sends the right messages to our bodies.
>
> In this easy-to-follow eight-week plan based on each individual's unique genetic needs, Dr. Hyman explains how to customize your personal weight-loss program with menus, recipes, shopping lists, and recommendations for supplements and exercise. Ultimately, you will rebalance and stabilize your metabolism -- an UltraMetabolism -- to maintain weight loss and enjoy lifelong health."
>
> – *Quoted from Amazon.com*

The 4-Hour Body: - *Timothy Ferriss*
An Uncommon Guide to Rapid Fat-Loss, Incredible Sex, and Becoming Superhuman

> Author Tim Ferriss is a bit of a Mad Scientist when it comes to weight loss and health. While I may have pricked my finger a few times to monitor the Insulin Rollercoaster, he had a glucose meter surgically implanted. He certainly takes this subject seriously and to the extreme.

Reading List

Change Your Brain, Change Your Body: - *Daniel G. Amen, M.D.*

Use Your Brain to Get and Keep the Body You Have Always Wanted

> We talked about brain and body chemistry being the key to living healthy. This book goes into exhaustive detail about the topic.

> "The key to a better body—in shape, energized, and youthful—is a healthy brain. Based on the latest medical research, as well as on Dr. Amen's two decades of clinical practice at the renowned Amen Clinics, where Dr. Amen and his associates pioneered the use of the most advanced brain imaging technology, *Change Your Brain, Change Your Body* shows you how to take the very best care of your brain."

> – *Quoted from Amazon.com*

Enter The Zone: - *Barry Sears, PHD*

A Dietary Road map

> "For years experts have been telling Americans what to eat and what not to eat. Fat, they told us, was the enemy. Then it was salt, then sugar, then cholesterol... and on it goes.

> Americans listened and they lost -- but not their excess fat. What they lost was their health and waistlines. Americans are the fattest people on earth... and why? Mainly because of the food they eat.

> In this scientific and revolutionary book, based on Nobel Prize-winning research, medical visionary and former Massachusetts Institute of Technology researcher Dr. Barry Sears makes peak physical and mental performance, as well as permanent fat loss, simple for you to understand and achieve.

> With lists of good and bad carbohydrates, easy-to-follow food blocks and delicious recipes, The Zone provides all you need to begin your journey toward permanent fat loss, great health and all-round peak performance. In balance, your body will not only burn fat, but you'll fight heart disease, diabetes, PMS, chronic fatigue, depression and cancer, as well as alleviate the painful symptoms of diseases such as multiple sclerosis and HIV.

> This Zone state of exceptional health is well-known to champion athletes. Your own journey toward it can begin with your next meal. You will no longer think of food as merely an item of pleasure or a means to appease hunger. Food is your medicine and your ticket to that state of ultimate body balance, strength and great health: the Zone."

> – *Quoted from Amazon.com*

NOTES

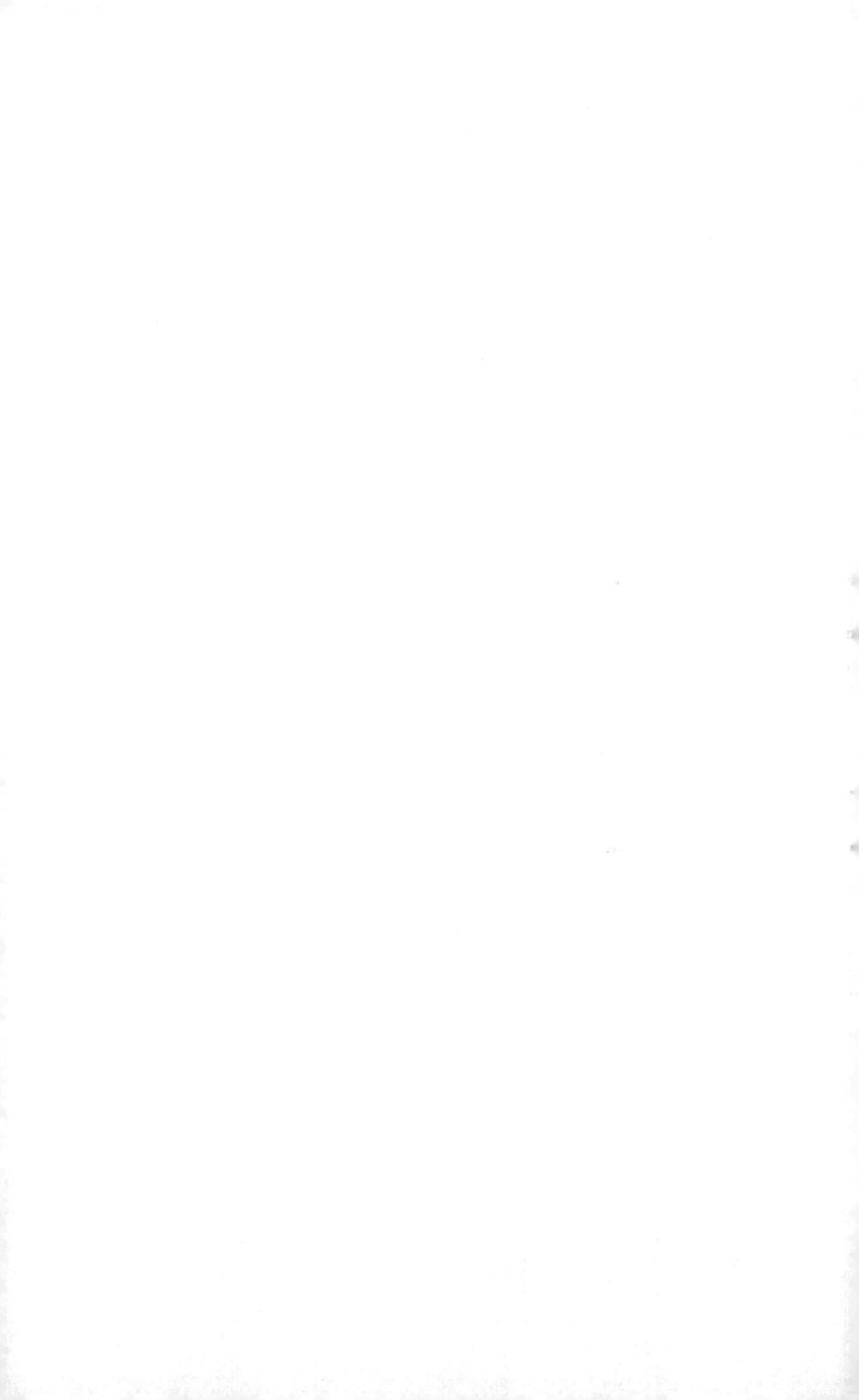

Made in the USA
Columbia, SC
10 June 2019